The Silent Pandemic

*Stories & Solutions First Hand Accounts
of Life with Opioid Addiction and
How to Find the Way Out*

**Recovery Connection Folks
Who've Been There Before**

Table of Contents

Introduction

Can You Help Me Sell Piss to Doctors?

Michael's Story

My name is Michael Brier and like so many millions of others, I started to use drugs and alcohol at a fairly young age. I was tall for my age, so when I was 18, I didn't have too much trouble walking into any liquor store with a fake id and buying cases of beer for my friends. We used to hang out down the street on the rock fencing of the boulevard and have a good time. I drank well before 18, though. When I was 13, I packed my trunk for overnight camp with a case of beer and shared it with everyone when I got there.

It took me a couple years before I transitioned into smoking marijuana. I had never been a fan of smoking since I had seen the damage it did to my grandmother, so I tried to stay away from it. However, peer pressure won, and I started smoking every day with my friends. As I did, I became more and more involved in the drug scene, using 'shrooms, hash, cocaine and my favorite drug of choice, acid. Lots of Grateful Dead concerts later, and I finished college, got married, had a child and built a business.

Over the next 30 years or so, I went back and forth between using and not using. I was running a multi-million-dollar business and eventually ran into trouble with the government. Not the local kind,

I mean the big bad federal kind. After thinking I was such a big shot, I was eventually sentenced to 27 months in Federal Prison.

Long story short, I served 30 months (yeah, more trouble) and even served 5 of those months in the "hole." Good times! When I was finally released, I was faced with the reality that being a convict and being in recovery has one big thing in common. . . STIGMA!

Ever hear someone say that they would never hire a convict? Heck, that question is even asked on job applications sometimes. On top of past convictions, you also may still have drug and/or alcohol issues. Great resume for a job!

So, I knew getting a job was going to be virtually impossible. The best-case scenario was to think up a business idea and try to make that work with no money while living off of food stamps.

My AHA moment came when someone approached me with a job offer. He asked, "How would you like to sell piss to doctors for me?" Boy, did that sound like a dream job. Ha! However, if you have nothing else to do with your life, you ask the obvious question in return, "What does that mean?" The answer was that he wanted me to find doctors in Florida who were treating people suffering from drug addiction and were prescribing Suboxone. I had no idea what that was, but I told him to let me do my own research about it, and I would let him know.

Well, what does any good businessperson do at this point? The answer is that they turn to what is now the 21st century's version of an encyclopedia (that actually was a thing back when I was young) and started to research anything and everything I could find out about Suboxone on Google.

I came to find out that while more and more people were dying from overdose deaths each year, there was a shortage of doctors willing to treat people in the addiction field. I also found out that the reason for this came back to that word again . . . STIGMA. Many doctors didn't want "that type of client" in their offices while they were treating their "regular" clients. I found that disgusting.

I decided that I didn't want to sell piss. I mean, who would? I was tired of trying to build a business to make money. I wanted to build a business for a mission. That was the beginning of Recovery Connection Centers of America (RCCA).

Finding My Way Out of the Maze

Regis's Story

My name is Regis Burlas. I am a physician and the president/chief medical officer of Recovery Connection Centers of America. If you are reading this, you or someone you know probably has or is currently suffering from the disease of addiction. I lost my uncle, mother and younger brother to this devastating illness, and yet I could not recognize my own issues. Alcohol and drugs became my lover and my best friend. My existence became defined as a journey into the depths of insanity, despair and hopelessness. My world did not recognize anything that was not centered around "Regis." Increased tolerance and withdrawal symptoms became my norm. I forgot what it was like to peacefully fall asleep since I passed out each night. No longer did I wake up rested; rather, I came to with pain, cramps, tremors, and only one goal -- to get more alcohol and drugs.

This disease is described as cunning, baffling, powerful, sophisticated, patient, progressive and too often, fatal. This disease talks to us and hijacks our brains. People and things that we used to enjoy are replaced by drugs and alcohol. Family, friends and jobs are forgotten. Personally, I lost my wife, job, life savings, self-worth and inner peace. I was alone and did not care if I ever woke up.

However, on Christmas Eve of 2012, my sponsor found me semi-conscious in my apartment and took me to a recovery center where my life began to change. I was finally ready to admit my powerlessness over drugs and alcohol and that my life was unmanageable. This is the first step as outlined in Alcoholics Anonymous – no matter which program you work for recovery, you must accept this and want to get help. My recovery path was not easy, and it was not without relapse. I listened to how others achieved and maintained a life of sobriety. I underwent counseling and was told I had to change everything but my hair color. The people, places and things that were associated with my using had to go. On April 15th of 2013 I had what I hope will be my last drink/drug. Recovery, as we have here at Recovery Connection Centers of America, involves all aspects of life – physical, mental, emotional and spiritual (which has a different meaning for everybody).

Here at Recovery Connection Centers of America there is hope. There are no judgements made. Compassion, listening and teaching what recovery truly means are embraced. So, if you or someone you know is lost in that maze of hopelessness and despair, please reach out. I have been in that maze before and know how to get out. A future of inner peace and happiness awaits.

What is RCCA's Mission?

Recovery Connection is a group of Outpatient Medication Assisted Treatment Offices (Suboxone/Sublocade) with locations in Rhode Island, Massachusetts and coming soon to all of the United States. Our mission is to expand services for those suffering from substance use disorder with personalized medication and counseling services in an outpatient setting. We want to treat our clients with empathy and respect. We want to break down STIGMA and tell everyone that they deserve to be treated with first-class care regardless of their background.

We could rant and rave about the STIGMA in our society when it comes to addiction. There are people who say they care about treatment for those suffering but aren't willing to actually do anything about it. People who are hypocritical and say, "not in my backyard," don't seem to have their patients' best interests at heart.

At Recovery Connection Centers of America, we are committed to expanding services and offices across this country. This past year alone has seen a rise of over 30% in overdose deaths, and that is why we have titled this book "The Silent Pandemic."

Purpose of this Book

To say that we are in an opioid crisis would be accurate since nearly 120 people die from opioid overdoses in the United States every day. Let's put this into perspective. Picture yourself in a football stadium filled with fans. Look around at all the filled seats because that is how many people will die from opioid overdoses in any given year.

In fact, this past year during COVID-19, the crisis has become worse. Government data shows that drug overdose deaths were up 30% in the pandemic year, and substance use disorder also increases the risk of contracting COVID.[1]

Greg Graustein, Chief Clinical Director of (RCCA), Regis Burlas, Chief Medical Officer of (RCCA), and Michael Brier, CEO of (RCCA) have put this book together to describe their philosophy on substance abuse treatment. It is their goal to shout from the rooftops louder than all the damaging and misleading information that is out there. With the amount of people suffering from opioid addictions only rising, this book was designed to help those of you participating in or thinking of participating in a substance abuse treatment *process*. Usually when something is described as a "process," you can be sure that it's not one-dimensional and may present some difficulties. This is in fact the purpose of this book, which is to help you navigate the confusing and sometimes contradictory information that is out there.

Quick word of warning: This is not a self-help book; rather, it is a companion guide for those who have a substance abuse issue and are looking for information on the treatment process, specifically medication-assisted treatment. This is also a useful tool for those friends and families of addicts who want to understand addiction and the treatment process in order to help a loved one on their journey.

As you read through this book, please reach out with any questions or concerns you might have about treatment. Even if you are not in our area, we are happy to try and help you search for a provider. In many cities, you can dial *211 or *311 for someone to help. Remember, if there is ever an emergency, call 911 immediately and save a life.

Recovery Connection Centers of America
www.drughelp.com
(877) 557-3155

Chapter 1
Deep Dive into Opioid Addiction

Nicole's* Story

I grew up believing the lies of addiction stigma: "Addiction only happens to bad people. If someone gets hooked on drugs, they can just decide to stop whenever they want. People who come from stable homes don't need to worry about addiction. Dangerous drugs are sold on the streets by scary-looking dealers."

Based on these lies, I thought I didn't have anything to worry about. After all, I wasn't abused as a child or abandoned by my parents. I got good grades in school, graduated from college (twice), landed a great job, and had a wonderful group of friends. I wasn't in danger of getting hooked on drugs, or so I assumed.

I started taking opioid painkillers for a legitimate injury. After my third refill of Vicodin, I noticed something. Despite very clear instructions to take one pill every four to six hours, taking two at a time gave me an intoxicating surge of energy. I felt like the Hulk. I'd wake up early on the weekends, down a few pills at one time and turn into a house-cleaning machine. When the energy wore off, I'd take a few more pills and get to work in my garden or hike a few miles.

What I didn't pay attention to — or maybe what I chose to ignore — was the increasing number of pills I needed to maintain my high. I went from taking two Vicodin at a time to eight at a time. I was running through a 30-day prescription in under a week.

---

* Name changed to protect privacy

Around the same time, stories began to hit the news about the rampant abuse of hydrocodone painkillers in the South. Suddenly, my doctor was hesitant to write prescriptions for medications like Vicodin, Lorcet, Lortab, or Norco. Instead, he suggested I try this new painkiller. He said, according to his pharmaceutical salesman, it wasn't nearly as addictive as Vicodin. That's how I was introduced to OxyContin.

In a matter of months, I lost my job, pushed all my real friends away, destroyed the tiny bit of trust my family had left in me, went into massive debt, and established a firm hate for myself. I no longer spent quality time with the love of my life and one remaining soul who still loved me without judgement — my dog, Barley. I was a shell of the woman I used to be. Every waking second of every day was consumed by one thing: avoiding withdrawal at all costs.

I didn't realize I'd set myself up for a battle — a fight where the winner takes all and the "prize" was my life. I eventually ran out of money and could no longer afford to feed my addiction. It was a fork in the road, and I had to make a decision. I could continue down the same path and end up in jail or the morgue, or I could finally admit I was in over my head and ask for help.

I chose to seek help. I had tried to quit pills on my own a hundred times — and I failed a hundred times. I just couldn't make it through the withdrawals. The physical part of withdrawal was horrible, but the mental torture was just as bad. Going through the same process one more time scared me to death. I could not fail again. I was sick and tired of being sick and tired. I wanted my life back, and I wanted to feel genuine happiness again. This time had to be different.

I'd somehow managed to get — and keep — a job waiting tables around this same time. A girl at work (who happened to be in early recovery) recognized all the signs of my addiction, and she asked if I'd considered trying Suboxone in an outpatient Medication Assisted Treatment (MAT) program. I'd never even heard of Suboxone or MAT, but I wanted to know more.

I read everything I could find online about Suboxone and the types of therapy used in MAT. It almost sounded too good to be true — medication to prevent the agony of withdrawal, counseling to uncover and address the root causes of my addiction, and treatment provided in an outpatient, office-based setting.

I had absolutely nothing to lose, so I made an appointment. And it was the best decision I have ever made. Up to the point of my first appointment, my mind was obsessed with avoiding the gut-wrenching withdrawal symptoms of opioid addiction. I had almost convinced myself that the Suboxone wouldn't work — that no matter what, I'd still find myself curled up in a ball on my bed sweating and freezing at the same time, running to the bathroom every five minutes, my bones aching with every step I took.

But once I started Suboxone, my whole mindset changed. Suboxone actually prevented the sickness of withdrawal and that amazed me. The absence of withdrawal symptoms allowed me the time and peace of mind to work through the events that sparked my addiction. For the first time in almost two years, I felt my own emotions instead of avoiding and numbing them.

I never felt high or impaired while taking Suboxone. Once the OxyContin fog lifted, my mind cleared up. I started making sober, informed decisions. I'll never understand why people say you can't be sober while on Suboxone. I also wonder how many of the people who perpetuate that stigma have personally used Suboxone to get sober. On the proper dosage and taken as prescribed, you don't feel mentally or physically altered in the slightest. Sure, the medication can be abused, but doesn't that apply to most things in life? Sugar can be abused. Love can be abused. Making money can be abused. Collecting stamps can even be abused. But if you're serious about getting sober, abusing your medication isn't in the game plan and it certainly isn't on your to-do list.

With the help of Suboxone, my fear turned into hope.

Once I opened up to my counselor, a floodgate of feelings poured out. I had to relearn how to sit with my own emotions and work through them in a healthy way. I had to stop blaming everyone else for the poor decisions I made. I had to make amends with the loved ones I had hurt — and I had to accept that some people weren't willing to accept or trust my apologies just yet. I had to take responsibility for my addiction and promise myself I would do whatever it took to succeed in recovery.

For me, one of the best things about going through a MAT program was the outpatient office setting. It gave me the ability to enter recovery while still living at home. I didn't need to pay thousands of dollars to move into a treatment center and put my life on hold for months.

I went to work every day, paid my bills, and took care of my responsibilities. I played an active role in my own recovery, and that gave me a sense of pride. My clinical support team set me up with the tools to live addiction-free, but at the end of every single day, it was up to me to do the work.

- Nicole P from Warren, RI

Opioid Addiction Crisis

Opioid addiction has been defined as the compulsive use of opioids despite negative consequences. They are a class of drug that includes prescription pain medications as well as illegal drugs like heroin. Some opioids can even be prescribed by a doctor to treat pain, but when they are misused or abused, it can lead to dependency or addiction.

With the number of people who have substance use disorders on the rise, opioid addiction has become a trend that has quickly transitioned into a crisis. At the time of this book's release, the country will still be slowly emerging from a global pandemic that rocked the nation and created widespread fear, uncertainty, and panic. With it came an unprecedented rise in the number of both new people who have substance use disorders and those relapsing in recovery.

The numbers are troubling and highlight the importance of what treatment centers like Recovery Connection are doing within their communities. According to the Center for Disease Control (CDC), 81,230 people died of drug overdoses in the 12-month period ending in May 2020, which is by far the largest number we've seen. Much of that rise has been attributed to COVID-19 and the difficulties that accompany trying to overcome an addiction during a global pandemic.

The impact of the pandemic is yet to be seen, but early projections are showing a range of 27,644 to 154,037 predicted deaths from drug overdose, alcohol abuse, and suicide in the next 10 years.[2] The pandemic also brought an increase in the use of fentanyl and methamphetamines. Fentanyl is an opioid that has seen significant increases, specifically as a street drug. It is 50 to 100 times stronger than morphine and has caused countless accidental overdoses and deaths. Methamphetamine usage creates a unique issue since there is currently no antidote for an overdose nor are there any medications approved by the FDA that can be used to treat an addiction to this substance.

Further research done by Millennium Health shows that the United States is currently in the third and potentially the fourth wave of the substance use crisis that is intricately connected to overdose deaths. The first wave was the introduction and increase of prescription opioid abuse; the second wave was heroin; the third was the synthetic opioid wave, which includes Fentanyl, and the fourth wave is looking like the impact caused by the growing use of methamphetamine.[3]

Opioid Addiction Causes and Symptoms

Opioid addiction can begin from the feelings of euphoria that come from the use of the drugs. Opioids can be incredibly addictive since they activate powerful reward centers in your brain. Once you take an opioid, it triggers the release of endorphins, which are your brain's feel-good neurotransmitters. This means that those endorphins are then able to reduce your perception of pain while simultaneously increasing your feelings of pleasure. For someone experiencing chronic pain, both emotionally and physically, this type of escape can be immensely and immediately addictive. After the effects of the opioid wear off, the user may feel compelled to revisit that high again even with the risk of long-term consequences.

The issue arises when the user continues to take opioids, whether prescribed or obtained illegally. With repeated use, the body slows its production of endorphins, meaning the user must increase dosage to maintain the intensity of their high. In many cases, users may turn from prescribed opioids to illegal drugs such as heroin and fentanyl, which is a drug laced with other contaminants that make it much more powerful than opioids. Extended use of opioids can lead to an addiction that can be hard to overcome, or it can also cause an accidental overdose.

Accidental overdoses happen more frequently than some might assume. Many times, this is in direct connection to those who isolate while using, which can be an excuse for some who may not identify their drug use as a problem because it is intermittent, which means they wouldn't consider themselves a "full blown addict." People who begin using drugs alone become comfortable taking the risk of hiding their behaviors. This is dangerous because if an overdose occurs, will anyone even know they are using? Also, over time, people become comfortable with using a certain amount of something, and then if they take a break from their drug of choice, they may not realize their tolerance for that substance has decreased. This means, if they use that same amount again, they can increase their risk for overdose.

To determine if you or someone you know has an opioid addiction, there are a number of symptoms that when displayed, indicate possible addiction to include: inability to control opioid use, uncontrollable cravings, drowsiness, changes in sleeping habits, weight loss, frequent flu-like symptoms, lack of hygiene, isolation from friends or family, stealing, financial difficulties, and decreased libido. For some, the addiction may have started after being prescribed the medication. But, even if the start of usage was medically conducive to recovery, dependence can lead to harmful addiction that can detrimentally impact the user. Being aware of these causes and symptoms will provide essential information for someone struggling with an addiction or friends and family of someone who starts presenting the symptoms of an addiction.

Addiction Demographics

The CDC doesn't keep track of overdoses in conjunction with race; however, extensive research is showing that Black Americans are suffering the most from this crisis. A study conducted in Philadelphia found that overdose deaths surged 50% in Black residents while among white residents, the numbers stayed relatively the same. A similar study conducted in California showed almost identical data. This isn't necessarily new information since health and social inequities have existed for years, but the pandemic served to highlight it more.

Not only are there disparities in fatalities in conjunction with drug addiction, but the data is also showing that treatment options are more readily available for whites while people of color regularly face arrest and incarceration, categorizing them as criminals. Within urban communities there is a noticeable lack of treatment options, which according to a study published in the Journal of the American Medical Association (JAMA), overdose deaths in those communities could be reduced by 40% within two years with viable and accessible treatment.[4]

The Need for Effective Treatment

To believe that the solution is simple would be minimizing the long-term effects that this crisis is having on individuals, families, and entire communities. With the amount of misinformation and organizations capitalizing off of this crisis, there is an ever-increasing need for effective treatment. And as we dive deeper into the core of addiction, it will be evident that there is need for a multi-dimensional treatment process. It's not a quick fix, and you will see this from the next chapter as we will dive into the "why" behind addiction.

Chapter 2
The Why Behind Addiction

Trish's Story*

Trish is a 31-year-old mother of two who is employed full time and also recently began taking Suboxone. A fall six years ago transformed her life from one of being physically active to one of constant pain. Her doctor prescribed opioids, including OxyContin and methadone to help her manage her intense discomfort. In September, she finally had surgery to repair her damaged hip, and after the surgery she worked hard to reduce her pain medications.

"I was so done with being sick all the time. I had taken prescription methadone before to manage my pain, but I didn't like the side effects. Also, since doctors need special authorization to prescribe it, I would have had to go to a different GP. So, I decided to try Suboxone."

She says her transition period was difficult, with 12 days of intense illness and three visits to the emergency room.

"I had long-lasting withdrawal symptoms, likely from being on opioids for six years, so my system just crashed."

After one month on Suboxone, things are looking up. She says she is still in pain, but she's focused on regaining her muscular strength through water-based exercise. Mentally, she says, it is a relief "not being stuck to planning your day around your pain meds." She had been taking medication every six hours to try

---

* Name changed to protect privacy

and balance out the highs and lows. But on Suboxone, she takes her dose at night before bed and says, "There are no side effects, like terrible night sweats or those hours before your next dose when you feel awful."

- Trish S Warwick, RI

Trauma and Addiction

The reasons behind addiction can be more complex than at first glance. Each individual has had different experiences and lingering trauma that may lead to them using to the point of addiction. Understanding the why behind addiction is essential for both the user and the professional treating the person.

Latent or past trauma can be such an integral aspect of addiction. For many, trauma occurs at a young age and can be repeated into adulthood. In fact, two-thirds of children in the US are exposed to trauma prior to the age of 16.[5] The trauma can range from abuse and community violence to family substance use and loss of a loved one. At such a young age, a child's emotional and physical development may be stunted, causing even more issues that manifest themselves as they grow older. For some, turning to addictive substances can then become the catalyst for coping with negative emotions that they have not been equipped to handle.

Additionally, in homes where the parental figures were either disconnected, unsupportive, or abusive, the children often do not learn positive strategies on how to cope with emotional issues. And for those who have suffered abuse, it can actually damage parts of their brains that control behavior and impulsivity.

With all of the intense aftermath that can come from childhood trauma, many turn to substances that can help numb the pain, both physically and emotionally. Research shows that one of the main reasons people self-medicate is to escape a certain situation, which makes sense when you consider that roughly 66% of opioid users suffer from some form of childhood abuse and around 60% of users suffer from some form of untreated psychological illness. In fact, one peer-reviewed study found that the more childhood trauma a person was subjected to, the higher the self-medicating dose of opioids was administered.[6]

These traumatic events are known to lead to Post Traumatic Stress Disorder (PTSD), which is common among individuals using opioids. In fact, opioid users have the highest rate of PTSD among substance users. When the trauma becomes deeply rooted within, it can display itself through emotional and behavioral problems, psychological disorders, and the inability to function in the day to day, which are then numbed through addiction.

A number of studies have been conducted on the connection between addiction and trauma. One such study that served to highlight the intricate connection between the two was conducted in 2013. Since research already shows that substances users are twice as likely as the general population to experience a traumatic event, this study showed even more relevant data concerning trauma histories that further explains the connection between addiction and trauma.

The study's participants were broken up into three different groups -- the first group was dependent on prescription drugs, the second on nicotine, the third on cocaine. Their trauma histories (general, sexual, physical, and emotional) were compared, and the results showed that all three groups showed high levels of trauma exposure. But what was the most revealing was the differences that arose with the data from those addicted to prescription opiates. From the responses provided, this group experienced a greater number of general and total traumas, and they reported a younger age of their first trauma.[7]

Understanding this connection between trauma and addiction is essential because until the "why" of an addiction is determined, the cycle will simply repeat itself. This is where counseling becomes such an integral part of treatment and recovery, which we will address further in upcoming chapters.

Boredom and Addiction

Boredom is underrated when it comes to someone struggling with substance use issues. Heck, boredom is boring for anyone. A non-addicted brain can take boredom and recalculate a path towards something exciting or fulfilling. But take a brain that is dependent on stimulation from substances and regularly seeking a high from pills or drugs, and boredom can feel depressing and create a magnified sense of isolation and loneliness. Isolation and loneliness can also magnify feelings of shame, which can lead to self-medication to alleviate the negative feelings that have ensued.

It seems like a simple answer to grab some pills or to get a fix from a substance that will bring the high feelings. Even the very act of taking pills gives the sensation of doing something, which is a way to cope with boredom. But boredom is like the cloak of invisibility. It's only a blanket of nothing covering up something that most people are unsure of how to deal with because they can't actually see what they feel, and they aren't even sure how to identify what they feel. This is why understanding boredom as a trigger is important and certainly something to be addressed with people who express it as a feeling or a concern.

In a similar nature, experimentation is to boredom what milk is to cookies. Many people, especially teenagers, are more willing to experiment when they are bored, and it's important to understand that experimentation is as dangerous as boredom. Once considered a normal rite of passage, experimentation is now considered more dangerous and complicated because people don't always know the exact recipe for what they're taking or what they're going to feel once they take it. If someone experiments with one pill and the result is that they feel better after taking it, then they are much more likely to take another one, and then another and so on. So, whether it was because of boredom or because someone wanted to just try it once, it is a potential recipe for long term disaster.

Addiction and Chronic Pain

When an individual is struck with unbearable pain that has proven untreatable by moderate measures, opioids may be prescribed. Opioids are actually recognized as necessary and legitimate agents to treat pain. However, even though there is a level of effectiveness that can benefit the user, the risks can outweigh the benefits with the potential of misuse, abuse, diversion, addiction, and overdose deaths.

The impact of chronic pain can vary, but based on the data, some people experience intense pain every day. The responses to the Functioning and Disability Supplement of the 2012 National Health Interview Survey led to estimates that 126.1 million US adults experienced some pain during the previous 3 months. And of those, 25.3 million adults suffered every day and 23.4 million reported "a lot" of pain.[8]

Even though it is clear that chronic pain is an issue in need of a solution, the numbers are showing an alarming number of patients having a negative experience with opioids. After reviewing 38 studies of opioid-treated patients with chronic pain found that misuse averaged between 21% to 29% and addiction averaged between 8% and 12%.[9] While opioids can bring a short-term alleviation for those dealing with chronic pain, the research is showing that the risk of addiction and misuse can create long-term devastation.

The Gender Difference and Addiction

The opioid addiction crisis impacts both men and women; however, based on numerous studies, gender has a correlation with the different experiences that men and women have reported. Women are more likely than men to suffer from chronic pain, which means their introduction to opioids is based in their need for pain relief. There is also evidence that shows women, who have been victims of violence and abuse may be at higher risk for chronic pain. Also, women are more likely than men to take opioids as a way to cope with negative emotions and pain.

In contrast, men are more likely to use illegal sources of opioids and engage in risker administration of the drugs to include increasing the amount used as well as ingesting it by crushing and snorting or injecting. Men are also more likely to die from an opioid-related overdose, with fentanyl being the common substance used. Even though differences are evident in usage trends and gender, the common denominator is the need for treatment and a full analysis of the core of the addiction for effective treatment methods.[10]

Chapter 3
The Destruction

Amanda's *Story*

I think 5th grade D.A.R.E. class piqued my interest in drugs. But if it wasn't that, then something caused me to be really curious, and I ended up reading all the books about drugs at my library. I was really drawn to the drug culture and my friends were a group of free thinkers, artists and musicians, so very few of them thought drugs were bad. I remember drugs were easily accessible and since I wanted to do them, I sought them out.

I was using hard drugs heavily for 15 years, and I have been hooked on Heroin for the last 3-4 years. I always viewed medicine for treatment and street drugs for getting high, so my addiction didn't stem from prescriptions at that time. I skipped the pharmacy altogether.

It all came to an end when I landed in jail and went through withdrawal for 24 hours before my dad bailed me out, as long I agreed to go to rehab. I was too exhausted, so I just gave in and spilled 15 years of secrets about my addiction to my mom and dad. It totally crushed them, and I didn't even realize that until years later. However, I knew that honesty was the only way to keep me from going back.

I do remember thinking at the time, "This is the end of my road." And if I admitted it, I didn't want to go through that again. Despite my thoughts, I still tried to leave rehab early, and when my ride didn't answer, that's when I finally accepted that I needed the help.

---

* Name has been changed to protect privacy

I think it was obvious I was struggling. I was no longer working; I was evicted twice in a row after paying rent for 12 years on my own; I often had the "flu"; I looked like crap; and I was being even more selfish and manipulative than usual. But I never told anyone I was struggling or that I wanted or needed help. I was far too confident while I was using to accept that things were out of my control.

I didn't have a choice about getting treatment and there weren't many options back then. My parents called my childhood best friend who is a social worker, and she gave them the state placement phone number. I literally went where they told me, but it really helped going to a MAT program where I was given Suboxone.

- Amanda F Attleboro, MA

The impact from addiction can be multi-faceted and complex. From mental, physical, emotional and relational consequences, a user's life may be completely out of control and almost unrecognizable from before they started using.

Physical Damages

The short-term effects of opioids are perhaps the main draw for continued use. When the user is able to escape their current reality to a pleasurable feeling of euphoria and drowsiness, they may be willing to risk long-term consequences. The truth is, the high is short-lived while the effects of nausea, vomiting, weakened immune system, slow breathing rate, coma, increased risk of HIV and hepatitis, hallucinations, collapsed veins, clogged blood vessels, and the risk of choking can be the long-term effects. Even when opioids are used for medical purposes, there are physical changes that can occur with the brain as well. Studies have shown significant size changes in several critical areas of the brain, even when patients take opioids as prescribed. These changes remained even months after patients discontinued opioids. The damage to the brain can impact mental functioning as well.

Mental Damages

Since opioids target the brain, there can be a significant amount of mental damage that can occur over time. Continued usage can cause drastic alterations to how the brain functions by creating neurological changes that alter the brain's reward system. This can cause the brain to go through extreme highs when the drugs are present, creating feelings of euphoria and pain relief, to the extreme lows of confusion and drowsiness. As the drug use continues, simple tasks may become more difficult and the brain's ability to handle day to day operations can diminish.

Mental health issues can arise as well since studies show that people addicted to drugs are roughly twice as likely to suffer from mood and anxiety disorders. It is estimated that 43.4 million (17.9 percent) adults ages 18 and older experience some form of mental illness. And of these, 8.1 million have substance use disorder. It is unclear as to whether the addiction caused the mental health disorder or vice versa, but there is a clear connection between the two.[11]

Emotional Damage

In many cases, individuals may start drug use specifically to avoid dealing with negative emotions. The reason for this is the feeling of euphoria experienced from drug usage can lessen or completely remove fear, anxiety, depression, sadness and other emotions that the individual may not be able to handle. The flip side of this is that those negative emotions the individual is trying to escape will intensify once the feeling of euphoria wears off after using the drug. One study revealed that long-term opiate use was found to alter blood flow between both hemispheres of the brain. When one hemisphere receives more blood than the other, some individuals reported that they experienced more negative moods while others reported intense mood swings with increased anxiety and depression.[12]

Relational Damage

One of the devastating aftermaths of addiction is the impact it can have on close relationships with friends, family and romantic partners. The reason for this varies based on the behaviors of the individual struggling with substance use disorder. According to the Bay Area Addiction Research and Treatment (BAART), there are 5 ways that opioids can impact relationships with loved ones. The first way is through deception since many individuals struggling with addiction may lie about their behaviors. The lies may start out as small and seemingly harmless, but as each lie builds, it creates a pattern of deception that gradually destroys trust. Loss of trust then becomes central to the slow eroding of the relationship because once trust is gone, it can be difficult to recover. This can be especially true if the individual struggling with the addiction steals from a loved one or continuously denies any strange behaviors despite evidence.

Another way that addiction can impact relationships is through potential violence and abuse that can be brought on by volatile behaviors due to mood changes or aggression from opioid use. Despite all of the turmoil, some loved ones may fall into the cycle of enabling because they are trying to help. However, enabling only allows the individual struggling with addiction to continue their opioid misuse. Enabling behaviors include taking over responsibilities at home, minimizing negative consequences of drug abuse, picking up their prescriptions, paying their bills, and making excuses for them. Finally, the relationship itself may become codependent as the loved one may find purpose in taking on the role of caretaker and enjoying the feeling of being needed.

Unfortunately, codependency can then make the relationship toxic for both parties involved.[13]

The impact of drug addiction can go far beyond just the physical damages that can be evident with the naked eye. Deeper damage that impacts individuals mentally, emotionally and relationally can push them into a state of depression, giving them a sense of hopelessness. And many times, that place of hopelessness can be the first step towards much needed change.

Chapter 4
5 Stages of Change

Robert's* Story

I'm a 46-year-old, divorced father with custody of my 6-year-old daughter and 7-year-old son. I have zero support from any extended family. For years I've relied on pills to get me through making dinner, doing dishes, house cleaning, laundry, homework, baths, cub scouts (I'm a den leader), girl scouts, modeling classes, and all the things that make up a family's life.

The guilt was horrible! Everybody else seemed to be able to deal with life, but I wasn't able to. I tried everything to stay clean: self-help books, meditation, religion, Native American wisdom, positive thinking, vitamin therapy, shamanism, counseling, NA meetings, a rehab stay, and the good ol' -- stand-by, white knuckle, skin of your teeth, cold turkey.

I quit for the 1000th time at the end of September for 1 week, for my daughter's birthday. I really wanted her to have her father back, clean. God, the shame of relapse! Everyone tells me I'm a great father and how my children are so lucky to have me. It would make me cringe to hear it. If they only knew how sad and pathetic I was without my Vicodin.

Anyway, the other day, for the first time in years, I picked up the kids after work and made dinner, took my daughter to modeling class, finished homework and ran baths — all without Vicodin! My energy level was high all evening and

---

* Name changed to protect privacy

not one single craving! No depression! I felt as if the weight of the world had been lifted from my shoulders.

*I felt great all the next day. Normal energy level, good mood, no headache or nausea. I took the kids to a roller-skating party in the evening, **all without Vicodin. All on one 8 mg dose of Suboxone at 8 am.** I just can't believe it!*

As we all snuggled in a chair reading a bedtime story last night, the relief I felt was overwhelming.

"Daddy, what's the matter?"

"Nothing, honey. Daddy's okay."

"Are you crying?"

"Yeah, just a little."

"Why, Daddy? Why are you crying?"

"I'm just so happy!"

"That's silly!"

"I know. I love you so much."

"I love you, too, and I'm happy, too!"

The fact I can stay "normal" by taking medicine is amazing. Being stable on 5 mg gives me hope for the future. I don't know if there is a "honeymoon period" with Suboxone, but I plan on being very careful of triggers in the coming weeks. Not only has Suboxone given me another chance at life, but it has also given my kids their daddy back.

- Robert N Taunton, MA

The Big Ask

At Recovery Connection, we often say that the hardest part of recovery is asking for help. You may know that you have a problem and can excuse it away in your mind for months, years, or even decades. But by seeking treatment, you are saying — most importantly, to yourself — that you have a problem you cannot fix on your own. It's a deeply personal problem, too. You've likely attempted to quit "cold turkey" in the past, either through your own determination or due to a lack of money or access.

The truth is, detoxing from substances is challenging, but nothing is more difficult than living a lifestyle that revolves around obtaining and using drugs. You may have relapsed a million times and found yourself in the freezing cold while cooking for your next hit. Not to mention, all the "close calls" with law enforcement and the need to always be on the lookout. You're most likely tired of being angry and resentful of the struggles you face on a daily basis.

If you have reached the point of wanting to get help, we are here to give you the answer to the question of where to find help.

Stage 1

Precontemplation

If you are reading this book for your own personal use, there is a good chance that you are already beyond the "precontemplation stage." This is the stage where an individual does not recognize that the consequences of their addiction are causing issues in their life.

When most individuals start with a new substance, they may only use it recreationally, on the weekends, or in small doses. This is the "honeymoon phase" of addiction. You may even have friends or loved ones comment that you seem more cheerful and the workday may go by faster. Not only that, but your work may also seem more enjoyable.

At the precontemplation stage of addiction, you will ignore the warning signs and refuse to recognize that the consequences you are facing are caused by the addiction itself. At this moment, you may or may not be in the "precontemplation stage."

Within the precontemplation stage, there are four categories – reluctant precontemplators, rebellious precontemplators, resigned precontemplators and rationalizing precontemplators. The reluctant lacks sufficient knowledge about the dimensions of the problem and the personal impact it can have. The rebellious is afraid of losing control and has a large investment in their addictive substance of choice. The resigned feels hopeless about change and the energy required to make that change. The rationalizing has all the answers and believes that others may have an addiction problem, but it is not really a problem for them.[14]

Stage 2

Contemplation

Once you move from the precontemplation stage, you enter contemplation, which is when you are able to acknowledge that you have a problem, and you start thinking about solving it. In this stage, you aren't essentially making plans yet. You don't have anything definitive; you just start wondering about possible solutions. This is where your thinking starts to become more futuristic in nature as opposed to focusing on the past. You may know the destination and even how you are going to get there, but you still aren't ready to go. There can be a mixture of activity, anxiety, anticipation, and excitement in this stage.

Stage 3

Preparation

In this stage, there are still a number of doubts and apprehensions present, which is why you might need more convincing. However, what makes this stage more hopeful is that you are planning to take action and are making final adjustments before you begin to change your behavior.

Stage 4

Action

At this point, you've started making behavior changes, modifying your surroundings, and maybe even checking into a treatment center or seeking an outpatient facility for assistance. This stage is one of the most difficult because it requires the greatest commitment of time and energy. But at this stage, change is most apparent to yourself and those around you.

Stage 5

Maintenance

While taking action is one of the most powerful steps in change, to believe that after action comes mastery is a dangerous mentality. Without a commitment to continuous maintenance, there can be relapse and a return to the earlier stages of precontemplation and contemplation. It is important to note that even if you reach the maintenance stage, it is common to go back to earlier stages again after a relapse. It is okay to understand that the stages of change aren't final or linear. After you embrace this truth, you can be patient with yourself and understand that change takes time and a commitment to the process while avoiding the ever elusive and unrealistic ideal of perfection.

It doesn't matter what stage you find yourself in, just know that each stage has value. The most important aspect of these stages is to progressively make your way to the point where you can start receiving the help you need. Though it may be difficult, once you finally reach the stage where you believe you can benefit from treatment, you are now able to look into your options to decide what will work best for you and your recovery process.

Chapter 5
Where to Look for Help

Laura's* Story

I come from a long line of drug users and alcoholics, so to say that it's in my genes is an understatement. I started using at a very young age. I was pulled in by the glamour of drug use. I started smoking pot and popping pills by the time I was 12. I was smoking pot with my dad by age 14 and doing cocaine with my mom when I was the ripe old age of 18.

*But it wasn't until I was 19 when I found my true downfall, **HEROIN**. I, unlike most people, didn't start with recreational use; instead, I dove in headfirst. Being a long-time addict already, there wasn't a lot stopping me. During the next 3 years, I was in an extremely abusive "drug-based" relationship, I lost a great job, lost some great friends, filed for bankruptcy, and most importantly, I lost myself. I hit a bottom low enough to leave that toxic relationship and check myself into a detox. I thought I was so fed up with the way I was living that I could do this on my own. I stayed clean for about 6 months. My relapse had nothing to do with willpower. I am an addict. I have a disease. I started to use pain pills again for recreation, somehow justifying, that because it wasn't heroin it was okay.*

I realized I couldn't do this on my own again. I checked myself back into a facility. This time with a new attitude and committing to a "real program." I started Suboxone and reluctantly going to Narcotics Anonymous (NA) meetings. Two days into my new program, I could feel myself changing. NA turned out to

---

* Name changed to protect privacy

be a lifesaver. I became the secretary at my home meeting, gaining strength from my elders and providing hope for the newcomer.

This time was different. After I left the treatment center, I didn't have the urge to use right away. Because of the buprenorphine, I learned there was a life beyond opioid abuse.

I have been on buprenorphine since October. I started at 16 mg a day for 10 months, now I take one 8 mg pill in the morning. I am anticipating celebrating 18 months clean and serene. I am now planning my wedding for September of next year with someone who doesn't use but does understand. I got another great job. I was super excited to (honestly) pass a drug test for the first time. One of my biggest achievements is that I am now able to plan a family of my own! Being an addict for literally half my life, I didn't think it would be possible to live drug free. Look out world, **here I come***!*

- Laura B Worcester, Ma

The Truth Sets You Free

Now that you've reached the point where you know you have a problem, you can start looking for help for your problem with substance abuse. If you're reading this and still don't think you have a problem, ask yourself if you can relate to any of the stories or the content from these pages. If you don't want to admit you have a problem, maybe you could ask yourself if your life is really going the way you want it to. Are there areas of your life that you know are holding you back, but you just can't seem to overcome them? Sometimes, it's important for all of us to take a moment of self-reflection where we can truly be honest with ourselves.

Once you get to the point of admitting that you need help, it can be difficult to know who or what to turn to for that help. It's great to have friends and family members on your side supporting you, but many individuals with a history of substance abuse have strained relationships with family and friends. The good news is that there is still help available to you even if those close to you aren't able to provide the support you need.

Substance Abuse and Mental Health Service Administration

One great place to start looking for help with your addiction is the Substance Abuse and Mental Health Service Administration's website - - www.samhsa.gov. On the SAMHSA website, the first link in the toolbar labeled "Find Treatment" will take you to several tools, including a substance use treatment locator, behavior health treatment services locators, buprenorphine physician and treatment program locator, as well as other locator tools that can help you get started on your path.

The SAMHSA website also features a national database of doctors and practitioners specializing in addiction recovery. Even in the small state of Rhode Island, the website lists over 50,000 practitioners. So, the chances of finding a substance use practitioner in your area are very likely.

The Internet

The internet can be a fantastic resource for seeking help. It's practically anonymous and allows you to conduct research that will help you narrow down your treatment options. No matter where you are in the world, as long as you have access to the internet, you can visit Google and type in the search phrase "recovery addiction treatment near me." The first treatment centers that will pop up will be paid placement (these have the letters AD next to the link). That means, the first result isn't always the best option. Look through the results and research the treatment center by reading reviews.

Consulting with Friends

Asking your friends about substance abuse treatment can be a double-edged sword. Most users surround themselves with other users, so if you are in a group that continues to use, these may not be the best people to ask for advice on treatment. Secondly, these same people, who likely do not want treatment themselves, may try to discourage you from seeking treatment.

If you are curious about the recovery process, you can reach out to people who are not users or people who are currently going through the recovery process. Either way, finding support from people who understand what you are going through based on their own experiences can be extremely helpful. At Recovery Connections, we have many new patients come through our doors because they were referred by friends or family members.

When you enter treatment, you will most likely be surprised at the number of people working in these centers who are former users. Some of the best people working in substance abuse treatment are former users who are looking to help others going through the process. Normally, people who have never done drugs before are not the kind of people you would typically ask about getting help with substance abuse.

However, if you are the person or the friend who is approached by someone seeking help, it's important to skip the judgement section of the conversation and skip right to this line: Repeat after me, "I'm proud that you are ready to change. Let's make a phone call and get you an appointment." It's actually that simple. It's not your job as a friend, family member or person of support to fix someone asking for help. It's simply your job to be their compass and provide direction so that they can find the resources they need. Don't complicate your support; the disease is complicated enough. Simply support their decision to get help and support the next step of taking action.

Chapter 6
The Ins and Outs of Treatment

William's Story

I got all the pills I could get out of my doctor for a period of 3 months. By that time, I was up to 20-25, 10 mg of Percocet a day. My wife has been a pain-management patient all of our marriage, and for all those years, I would never touch her medicine because she truly needed it. After I became addicted, I lost control and began to take her drugs to keep the withdrawals away. This went on for about a year.

Then, I found what I thought was a friend who kept me supplied for the next year, but the cost was killing us financially. I tried many times to wean down but never got very far. The times I would run out were like living a nightmare. It was awful. By this time, I was up to about 200-250 mg of Oxycodone a day. I would even wake up at night and need to dose so I could go back to sleep. I always hated that because I felt like I was wasting the drugs. I had more wean-down sheets than you could imagine. I tried everything.

Then, during a family reunion, I told an uncle about my back pain and asked him for some pills. He was a Vietnam vet who got blown up in Nam. He had all the drugs you could imagine and rarely took them, so he started supplying me with 40 mg tablets of OxyContin. I didn't chew them at first. Then, I figured out that they worked better if I chewed 2 or 3 at a time. This went on for another 6 months, but at least I wasn't paying for the pills. They were free to me. Then, I told my uncle

_____

* Name changed to protect privacy

the truth about my back and the fact that I was severely addicted to opiates. He had what I thought was my answer — methadone. It did stop my withdrawal, but within a year, I was doing an average of 80 mg per day. I always took enough to get high, and when I would build a tolerance, I would keep increasing. This whole time I told my wife I needed pills for my back so I could work.

On the first of March, my uncle passed away, and I was faced with no supply. I tried desperately to wean down again, but it didn't work. I prayed so many times for God to deliver me from this horrible addiction. I went to a methadone clinic for help. At this time, I just wanted to be under a doctor's care. I was afraid I would die sooner or later. The clinic wasn't taking any more patients, but they did tell me about a medicine called Suboxone and a doctor who would see me. I went home and called him, and to my surprise he actually talked to me that day. He said I was on too high of a dose to switch to Sub, but I told him I would do whatever it took.

He set up an appointment 3 days later. I did everything he said, even though I thought I would die. I was sick as a dog for a couple days. I showed up for my appointment 2 hours early that day and had every withdrawal symptom there is. I had lost 10lbs leading up to my appointment. He started my first dose at 4 mg, and I felt nothing. Then, he gave me another 4 mg and still nothing. When we got to 16 mg, I still felt bad but told him I was ok. After I got home, I called and took another 8 mg. I stayed on 24 mg the first week of treatment.

I am approaching 3 months on Suboxone, and I have my life back. I've successfully dropped down to 12 mg a day. I wish I would have found Suboxone a lot sooner, but I'm not a computer person so I had no way to discover it other than God answering my prayer.

- William D, Dedham, MA

What it's Like Going Through Drug Treatment

When you consider the potency of the drugs that are on the streets these days, the difficulty of treatment pales in comparison to the damage done to the body through addiction. Fentanyl, a synthetic opioid, is 10,000 times stronger than morphine (by volume). Even worse, there is a new drug known as carfentanil, which is 100 times stronger than fentanyl. These dangerously addictive substances and others like them are increasing in usage while the death rate continues to climb. And while users may struggle to get to the point of seeking treatment, there has never been a better time to have comprehensive and effective treatment available.

You may be ready to start exploring your treatment options but feel apprehensive because of the narrative you have heard about the treatment process. We wanted to provide you with as much information as possible so you can enter treatment more aware of what the experience will look like.

Everyone involved with this book has abused opiates and other drugs at one time. One thing you'll never hear us say is, "We beat it. We're done with it, and we'll never do it again." By recognizing that drug addiction is a lifelong battle, we are mindful to not let our guards down. There are many people in drug treatment that will say, "I wish I could go back to the way things were before I became involved with drugs." But, what those in recovery should really be aiming for is a new and improved life. Why go back to the old? We know where that path leads.

In writing this book, our greatest hope is that it will give you a realistic perspective of the treatment process. Once you arrive at a place of stability, you may even consider becoming a mentor to others. It's not only a great way to help those in need, but it's also a way to remind yourself of where you've been.

Types of Treatment

Probation-Mandated Treatment

There are many individuals who walk through our doors, not by their own choosing, but as stipulated by their probation agreement. To those we say, keep an open mind. We know in all likelihood that you would rather not be entangled with the criminal justice system, and you might prefer to keep living your life, using. Most likely, this is your first offense. But, even if the law doesn't catch up to you, life will. By that we mean that if you continue to use hard drugs, you may eventually find yourself up against mounting psychological, family, and financial issues. Give treatment a fair shot.

Long-Term Residential Treatment

This type of treatment provides 24-hour care and is not in a hospital setting. The best-known model for this is called therapeutic community (TC) with stays ranging from 6-12 months. The focus of this type of treatment is "resocialization" which strives to utilize the program's entire community to include the other residents and staff as active components of the treatment. The purpose of the treatment is to develop personal accountability and responsibility as well as training individuals to live socially productive lives. During the process, patients are encouraged to identify and confront destructive behavioral patterns and damaging beliefs that have kept them in a cycle of drug abuse. Many TCs also offer more support services like employment training that prepare the patient to reintegrate into society in a healthier manner.

Short-Term Residential Treatment

These types of programs are shorter but also more intense with a modified 12-step approach. The model consists of a 3 to 6-week hospital-based, inpatient treatment phase followed by outpatient therapy and participation in a self-help group such as Narcotics Anonymous (NA). The treatment following the inpatient care is highly encouraged since it is shown that after care programs reduce potential relapses from occurring.

Outpatient Treatment

These programs are more cost efficient than the other treatment options mentioned, and the types and intensity levels may vary based on the facility. Outpatient options are more suitable for individuals with jobs or extensive social support. Many outpatient facilities provide group counseling and services that are comparable to residential programs as well, which can be highly effective. At the same time, it's important to do your homework with these facilities because some may just offer little more than drug education.

Personalized/Group Drug Counseling

Addiction counselors have shown a positive impact on rehabbing and reintegrating drug users back into society no longer addicted to harmful substances. Through counseling, people who have substance use disorders can connect with a peer discussion group to promote a drug-free lifestyle and to create positive connections with others trying to get clean. Individualized counseling also helps people who have substance use disorders create short-term goals and coping strategies to abstain from drug use and maintain abstinence.

Inpatient v. Outpatient

All treatment programs can be divided up into two groups: inpatient and outpatient.

Inpatient

In an inpatient scenario, you are basically in need of immediate help. When you check yourself in for inpatient treatment, the staff is going to assess how you're doing physically and mentally. Then, they are going to create an action plan.

The first step is to do a physical checkup to make sure your body is not in -- or entering -- a shutdown. During this phase, the nurses and doctors will look at how stabilized your condition is and determine whether or not you have been using drugs or alcohol.

One of the problems opiate users have when going to an inpatient treatment program is that they are going to go through withdrawal symptoms including weakness, vomiting, "chicken skin," discomfort, etc. Some facilities prescribe medications to help them feel more uncomfortable while others do not. Once you've gone through the withdrawal state, then the medical staff can begin evaluating you to see what medications will help you regain some of your comfort.

If you have underlying medical conditions on top of your addiction, you will most likely be better off going into a hospital setting. The reason for this is, they have housing, counseling, a calendar of events to help give you structure, as well as nurse practitioners and nurses that can medically evaluate you to see if you're okay.

These inpatient stays can be short (from a hospital standpoint), but it all really depends on your level of addiction and what symptoms you exhibit during the detoxification process. For example, someone who's having an issue with opiates could be checking into an inpatient facility for two or three days. However, once they get started on a buprenorphine treatment, they can begin outpatient treatment.

If someone is detoxing from alcohol, usually it's a minimum of 5 days for that individual to go through the detox process to ensure they are physically and mentally cleared before they are released. Someone who is heavily dependent on alcohol can experience delirium tremens (DT). DT can actually harm you -- maybe even kill you. In an inpatient setting, if you do go into DT, the facility will at least have resources, staff, and medications available to make the symptoms less severe (and less lethal). Lorazepam and chlordiazepoxide are two types of benzodiazepines that are useful in treating DT.

Detox Centers

An example of an inpatient facility would be detox centers and facilities that exist to get you started with the treatment process. They essentially help you through the detox phase, but you will likely need to go through additional treatment, such as another rehab center. Detox facilities make sure the body has stabilized. Then they may refer you to another longer-term care plan or even a housing unit with just people in recovery. These provide an environment that is drug-free and houses people that are going through the recovery process. These types of centers can be found in just about every community.

Detox centers are actually a great way to connect with inpatient services and long-term care facilities. They can match your insurance or ability to pay with service providers in your area. These centers often have care coordinators that will match you and give you the support you need to further your treatment.

Outpatient

Outpatient centers typically rely on counselling and medication assistance, but someone may also be referred by their physician. Sometimes it's a case of a patient asking their doctor to be prescribed more opiates such as Vicodin. The doctor may refer them to a methadone or a Suboxone clinic to help them transition away from more addictive opiates including fentanyl, OxyContin, Vicodin or any other opioid drug.

Here are some examples of outpatient treatment options:

Rhode Island Model

The Rhode Island Model was established years ago in Rhode Island by Jim Gillen who is the Director of Anchor, which is a federally funded clubhouse model. In 2008, he joined Providence Center and helped create what's called Anchor Recovery Center. With funding through state and federal grants, he was able to create this Care Coach Recovery Center, which essentially promotes clients helping clients. He started this concept offsite from a mental health agency. He then joined forces with the events committee for the National Recovery Month. At a day long event, he opened a table on one small street in Providence where people could congregate to meet each other.

Over 300 people attended that first event. By 2013, that same event in Providence was attended by 15,000 people. State and federal politicians showed up, which gave Jim a platform to promote the care coach model. He then asked the federal government for funding to get care coaches 40 hours of training that would allow them to be certified and reach further into the community. His request was granted. After that was established, his model has spread throughout

New England with the hopes of bringing the success of this concept to other states as well.

Gillen's community clubhouse model focuses on people in recovery living with other people in recovery as they support each other through the process. So, within the same building, you would have housing but also a meeting space. In previous models, you would have a "big brother" or "big sister" that would sponsor you through the recovery process, but in the Rhode Island Model you have an entire community of people supporting you.

With this model, you are appointed a licensed and trained care coach who becomes your advocate. Let's say a person is revived with Narcan. There are many care coaches that will visit the hospital and coordinate care and help the individual get the treatment he/she needs. There are only a handful of states that have this model currently, but this type of recovery model is expected to expand.

How does this model compare to AA or NA?

Historically, the Narcotics Anonymous (NA) and Alcoholics Anonymous (AA) models would have someone that has been in recovery for at least a year or two who would act as a mentor for someone new to the program. Whether you call it a "big brother," "big sister" or "coach" is irrelevant; that person is there to pick up the phone and mentor the new member and be an advocate if they are thinking of using again. Both NA and AA follow the 12-step program that incorporates weekly meetings for accountability purposes.

Unfortunately, many NA programs are not that proactive when it comes to people who are in recovery and are using methadone, Suboxone, or some other type of Medication-Assisted Therapy. Some chapters of NA are so old school that they see Medication-Assisted

Therapy as a crutch. The coaching model doesn't adopt this mentality. In addition, the coaching model takes on a more personalized approach and the coaches must go through a certification process. This can mean the person struggling with substance use disorder will have a trained and certified advocate on their side to help them through recovery.

Sober Houses and Recovery Houses

There is one good recourse that is worth mentioning, even if it is not free per se, and that is a sober house or recovery house. A sober house is a place where a group of people are working toward recovery in a communal setting. It's sort of like having a family there to support you. Most of these programs are subsidized. So, while they may not be free, they will only cost you somewhere in the neighborhood of $150 to $175 per week, which may be too much if you are already paying rent at another property. While at a sober house, you will regularly undergo urine screens. This is to make sure that you are complying with the rules of the program.

Options for Payment

Insurance

While it may not be ideal, much of the care you receive might be dependent upon the insurance you have. As a rule of thumb, commercial insurance has a tendency to open more doorways. Treatment facilities favor major insurance providers like Aetna, Blue Cross, Cigna, United, etc. Also, if you're under the age of 26, then you likely still have coverage under your parent or guardian's plan.

Having commercial insurance usually means that you have better options, facility-wise. This may be a facility that is a little bit more private or independent. If you don't have commercial insurance, there's not too much to worry about. You might miss out on better meals and more treatment options, but not having commercial insurance isn't a deal-breaker.

Employee Assistance Programs

If you are employed with a medium- to large-size organization, there is a good chance that they have an Employee Assistance Program (EAP). Employee Assistance Programs are voluntary, work-based programs that provide free confidential assessments, short-term counseling, medical referrals, and follow-up services to individuals who are experiencing personal and/or work-related issues. EAPs exist to help employees overcome addiction, mental health issues, grief, family issues, substance abuse, and psychological disorders.

EAP counselors work in a consultative role with managers and supervisors to address employee and organizational challenges and needs. Many EAPs are active in helping organizations prevent and cope with workplace violence, trauma, and other emergency response situations. To find your agency's EAP administrator, the work/life contact tool is available at:
http://apps.opm.gov/CCLContact/index.aspx

Medicare and Medicaid

The enrollment process and eligibility for Medicare and Medicaid are different in each state. The first step would be to call your state Medicaid program to see if you qualify and then learn how to apply. In some states, even if you have too much income to qualify, you can "spend down" to become eligible. The "spend down" process lets you subtract your medical expenses from your income to become eligible because you're considered medically needy.

You May Qualify for Disability

Quite a few people who have substance abuse problems also have a history of medical problems. For Medicare, you might be classified as disabled for Social Security purposes. You also might be able to receive disability insurance payments each month while also qualifying for Medicare coverage. Most people find that Medicare is well worth it, and the coverage for substance abuse treatment is much more affordable compared to a commercial insurance provider.

Being disabled doesn't mean you will have a lifetime disability. But, if you are going with an Affordable Care Act (ACA) plan, you should know that the enrollment period is only open for a brief time each year. Although, if you happen to lose your job or you are faced with some other type of adversity, they are usually willing to work with you. Each state will be different, so it's important to get as much information on this as possible to see if you qualify.

What if You Just Have Medicaid or Medicare

Long-term care can be quite expensive, but even if you only have Medicaid or Medicare, you still have housing options. There are many generous people who have gone through the treatment process and decided they want to open their doors to those in recovery. Some of these will rent you a room, whereas others might get financial support from the government, therefore making the treatment much less expensive.

Free Resources to Help with Drug Abuse Treatment

Fortunately, for many people who are looking to stop abusing their drug of choice by going the buprenorphine/Suboxone route, there are plenty of free healthcare options available. If you need help signing up for free healthcare, it's managed by the individual states, so you should get in touch with your state's department of health. Most of these websites are called "Health Source." They all work a little differently, but the point is that if you are low-income, you can get free insurance that will help cover the costs of treatment. Even if you make a lot of money, you will be richer once you are able to stop using illicit drugs.

Of course, when you sign up for health insurance, there is a lot of government bureaucracy to sift through and the process is slow. The hardest part of the application process is usually the waiting. You might have to wait up to three hours to reach someone on the phone, so that is something you will have to plan for. But beyond the wait, the interview process is fairly straightforward.

If you do qualify for free or reduced health coverage, you can expect to get a call each year to make sure you still meet the eligibility requirements for the program. You will also want to select a plan that covers the type of medications you will be on. Most medication-assisted therapy programs fall under a category called "sub-medic behavioral health counseling services."

Opiate dependency treatments are covered by the parity clause since the Affordable Care Act (Obamacare) forced all insurance companies (commercial, governmental, etc.) to cover addiction treatment.

Chapter 7
The Right Treatment Model for You

John's* Story

Not needing to go too far back, I had been taking some form of narcotics for the last 10 years. Fifteen years prior to that, I generally took narcotics only on occasion and mostly for recreational purposes. I don't believe during those years I was dependent on narcotics beyond my desire to "catch a buzz" or whatever. But, in 1998, I became a Christian and pretty much quit drinking, smoking and doing any kind of drugs whatsoever. Praise God, He gave me the strength to be successful, as I would end up being diagnosed with leukemia a few short years later.

The type of leukemia I had was AML (Acute Melogenic Leukemia). Without going into great detail of the actual treatment, I ultimately underwent extensive chemotherapy and finally the bone marrow transplant. I give the Lord all the credit for my survival and for providing me with wonderful doctors and caregivers. This disease was undoubtedly the most difficult challenge of my life.

I had so much to live for with two wonderful daughters, 6 and 11 years old, and a beautiful and faithful wife of over twenty years at that time. Fighting and surviving leukemia would turn out to be a journey that I would wish on no one, and yet one that I am thankful for having taken. Throughout my treatment, there were many opportunities to share the Lord with others and to build and improve my relationship with God. For that I am truly blessed.

---

* Name changed to protect privacy

In 2014, I moved my family to Fred Hutch Research Institute in Seattle, Washington in preparation for my BMT (Bone Marrow Transplant), which required full body radiation on top of chemotherapy. All in all, I was in the hospital for over twenty weeks, receiving my new bone marrow as the hope for saving my life. Although my bone marrow transplant was very long and difficult, it was also successful. But, because of having an unrelated BMT donor, I ended up getting GVHD (Graph vs. Host Disease) and having to take, for an extended period of time, high doses of the wonderful steroid called Prednisone. This drug helped to save my life, but in the process, it destroyed both of my hips and severely damaged one of my shoulder joints.

Within a year or so of my transplant, I had one hip replaced in January and the other in July of that same year. During the two years prior to my hip replacements, had it not been for various pain medicines, I would have been in a wheelchair because of the excruciating pain I was going through.

I admit that I have always liked the way narcotics made me feel, but during my leukemia and hip replacements, I actually had a legitimate reason for taking them. After bi-lateral hip replacement surgery, getting prescriptions for narcotics was not much of a problem, especially with my medical history. I of course, started sampling various pain meds such as Oxycodone, Dilaudid, Morphine, Ultram, and Demerol; finally settling on Norco 10's.

For me, the Norco was a perfect fit to not only help me deal with chronic pain, but they also made me feel better mentally. I have to say that many of my doctors, though willing to write me prescriptions, also gave me multiple warnings about becoming dependent on narcotics. Having had so much experience with surviving leukemia, I told them I was fine and able to discipline myself to using only the prescribed amounts. And for a few years, that was true. However, with me it's always been, if a little is good, more is better. Consequently, over the last five years, I started increasing the amount of Norco in order to get the same effects as when I first began. In the end, I was taking as much as 20 to 30 Norco 10's per day. Obviously, I had to source them through other means than legitimate prescriptions.

Four weeks ago, by the grace of God, I happened to hear on the radio about a website that said that they help people deal with narcotic dependency. As it turned out, the information I found on the SAMHSA website changed my life. I knew that I had a serious problem of dependency, as I had tried to quit on several occasions over the last few years with no success. Every time I tried to cut back on the Norco, I became so severely ill that I knew there was no hope for me. I once tried to quit "cold turkey" and became so sick that I thought I was going to die. I knew that I could never quit on my own.

I had admitted to my wife a year earlier that I had a narcotic dependency problem, and I began counseling to deal with some of the underlying reasons for my drug problem. However, I did not let her know the seriousness of my problem and ended up telling her that I had quit, when in fact I had not. Now I was really in trouble in that I could not take time off from work for treatment nor could I continue to take such large quantities of the Norco because it was, and had for years, been affecting my relationships with my family as well as others.

Overall, I lived a very successful life externally, but internally I was a mess. I nearly destroyed my marriage, severely damaged my relationship with my daughters, and was continuing to have to lie in order to obtain the narcotics that my body absolutely needed to feel normal; that is, without severe pain. Finding this website and reading about buprenorphine/Suboxone treatment was the beginning of seeing hope for myself.

I immediately began to read all of the educational information and literally every post that others had entered on the website's discussion board. I had a difficult time believing what I was reading. It was so encouraging to read about the success of so many people dealing with the same problem that I had. It was also great in understanding about narcotic addiction and dependency and realizing how many others there are who need treatment. But because of the stereotype and biases of many people, it is difficult to even find out, much less locate a facility that deals with buprenorphine/Suboxone treatment. For the size of the city I live in, there are only a few doctors willing to treat narcotic dependency with this medication.

Within two days, I had located Recovery Connection that offered the Suboxone treatment. I scheduled an appointment for the next day even though I was scared about making the commitment so quickly. That was the beginning of 2018. Although my doctor is a no-nonsense type of person, he is also one who is knowledgeable and very interested in helping people break their narcotic dependency, especially those who are genuinely interested in getting off of narcotics. I can say that I have not had one craving or desire to take any narcotics since I started taking Suboxone. The withdrawal symptoms are non-existent, with the exception of a little nausea. I am currently in counseling and taking it one day at a time.

- John P Boston, MA

When it comes to the different types of treatment options, it is clear that there are a number of choices that you have in front of you as well as payment options. But before launching into a treatment type, it is beneficial to look at one of the most effective models that is being used and the reason for its success.

Medication-Assisted Treatment (MAT)

Generally, the Medication-Assisted Treatment model has had impressive results and has actually become the gold standard for modes of treatment. At Recovery Connection, we've focused most of our efforts here and have seen so many success stories, which have been featured at the beginning of each one of the chapters in this book.

What is Medication-Assisted Treatment (MAT)?

Medication-Assisted Treatment (commonly abbreviated as MAT) combines three modalities: medication management, behavioral therapy, and counseling. The goal is to treat the chemical, social, and psychological effects of addiction in a comfortable office setting in order to build a sustained recovery process.

There are currently three FDA-approved medications on the market to treat opioid dependence. These are buprenorphine (commonly known by the trade names Suboxone or Sublocade), methadone, and naltrexone. These drugs have a solid track record for safety.

Why MAT?

Hundreds of peer-reviewed studies have proven the effectiveness of Medication-Assisted Treatment. At Recovery Connection, we believe this form of treatment gives the patient the dignity and respect they deserve during what is likely one of the most trying times of their life. The withdrawal symptoms experienced without assistance from medication can be intense and potentially dangerous. However, with the assistance of medication, studies have shown that the risk of relapse decreases significantly; it can stave off infectious diseases like HIV and it can prevent overdoses.

How Can it Help Me?

Medication-Assisted Treatment has two basic components: medication assistance (obviously) and counseling. MAT uses a partial opioid to block opioid receptors. The philosophy of MAT is that patients do not need to experience withdrawal (the cravings, irritability, insomnia, stomach pain, brain fog, diarrhea, vomiting, tremors, etc.) in order to overcome addiction. Addiction is bad enough. Why would you want to subject yourself to the full impact of withdrawal in order to get clean?

How Does it Work?

There are several components to Medication-Assisted Treatment. For one, there's the medication Suboxone (buprenorphine), which works by activating the opioid receptors without creating a high. The

MU receptors in your body that accept opiates become dependent on you adding an opiate to it. When it doesn't have one, it starts the process of withdrawal symptoms in the body. Regular opiates stay on the receptor 2 to 6 hours and fall off, creating a craving.

Buprenorphine is a partial opiate that fits the MU site, and it stabilizes it without creating a high. The real bonus is that it will stay for over 32 hours or more on the site, maintaining stability. Most importantly, if the MU receptors are really full and you then attempt a full opiate, it should block the majority of the effects.

But also note that this is a "medication-assisted" type of treatment, meaning the medication is only the medical approach to stabilizing from withdrawal and cravings. Recovery is what you do to pick up the pieces of what you have lost. That is why counseling is very important.

Benefits of Medication-Assisted Treatment

With Medication-Assisted Treatment, such as Suboxone therapy, you are actually taking a partial opiate to help with cravings and the symptoms of withdrawal. Programs such as Narcotics Anonymous are more puritanical in nature. They see treatment as avoidance, whereas a center such as Recovery Connections is more realistic. No one wants to go through the symptoms of withdrawal or cravings.

There is value in going through cravings and the sickening withdrawal phase, but there are many people who simply can't put their life on pause for a week or more as they go through detox. For this reason, buprenorphine, Suboxone therapy, and Medication-Assisted Treatment are now considered the standard in the field of addiction therapy.

Obviously, medication is a part of medication-assisted treatment (or MAT). This may sound counterintuitive or that patients are simply trading one substance for another, but Medication-Assisted Treatment is seen as an effective transition between use and non-use of illicit drugs such as opioids.

But MAT is more than just treating patients with medication. Medication-Assisted Treatments also include counseling and behavioral therapies. Medication-Assisted Treatment has shown to be effective in treating opioid use disorders (OUD).

The FDA has approved buprenorphine, naltrexone, and methadone for treating opioid dependence because these medications have proven to be effective and safe when used as directed.

How Long Does MAT Last?

Like other forms of treatment, there is not a set timeline in which patients should complete Medication-Assisted Treatments. As a MAT patient, you will be periodically re-evaluated to determine the need and effectiveness of the treatment.

Why We Recommend MAT

At Recovery Connection, we utilize Medication-Assisted Treatment because it fulfills a number of requirements. These include:

- Backing by scientific studies

- No legal constraints

- Less potential for stigmatization

- Treatment is focused on the patient

- Success rate is higher compared to other forms of treatment

Availability of MAT

One of the great things about centers such as Recovery Connection is that we make it a point to be ready for patients when they have their "aha" moment. Even after an overdose or some other adverse event, it can be so easy to start using again, especially when there is a one to two-week wait period for treatment.

Most of the time, when a person raises that perceived 10,000-pound phone, they are wanting help immediately. They may even subconsciously realize that the longer they wait to begin treatment, the more likely it is that they will begin using again. The person seeking help is usually ready to get started right away -- today or tomorrow. Recovery Connection and other medication-assisted programs can see patients either the same day or the next day. If you are in need of help, you usually don't want to wait longer than 48 hours. This is seen as a reasonable timeframe for someone who is looking to begin treatment.

It's worth noting that the first facility you select may not be the right one for you. There are thousands of treatment centers that focus on a core set of modalities. The good news is that if you do find that a certain program isn't meeting your needs, then you can at least better focus on what it is you are looking to get out of a treatment program. In other words, it's a jumping off point.

Call Recovery Connection

If you would like more information and advice on selecting a treatment center, you can reach us at 1-877-557-3155. Even if we're not in your area, you can still call and talk to us.

The Right Treatment Center for You

Is there such a thing as "the right" or "perfect" treatment center? It all comes down to personal preference. Whatever method you feel will best help you to get clean and remain clean will be the best option for you. Whatever takes you from Point A to Point B is the right plan for you. If you find that riding the teacup ride at Disney World is the best method for defeating your addiction, then by all means, do it. Whatever takes you from that point of craving and addiction to a place where you are happy and have shielded yourself from the possibility of relapsing is what you should continue to pursue.

As you consider your options, two questions you should ask yourself are: "Will this treatment match my needs?" and "Does it provide regular counseling?" If the answer is yes to both questions, then you may have found the right treatment for you. Remember, this is your treatment process, so take the time you need to do research and figure out if the treatment type, facility, and modality all work for you.

Chapter 8
Deep Dive into MAT

Ashley's* Story

I'm 30 years old, married with one child, and I'm a stay-at-home mom. I am addicted to hydrocodone, and I will be for the rest of my life. I took my first Vicodin about 5 years ago for back pain. I did not abuse it right away, but I did notice how much I liked the way they made me feel. I didn't even use them on a regular basis. About 6 months later, I had surgery to get breast implants, and it was very painful. The doctor gave me 60 pain pills. I started feeling better but kept on taking the pills anyway. And from that point on, I never stopped. As time went on, my tolerance got higher and higher, and before I knew it, I was taking anywhere between 20-30 of the 7.5/750 mg Vicodin.

During this time, I began to isolate from my friends and family. I lied to everyone. I was the head of the PTA at my child's school; I was taking karate lessons; I volunteered; and I was a part-time student. I slowly quit doing all of it because the pills were more important to me. I was a very active mom, always hosting sleepovers and play dates, and I became the druggie mom on the couch that just wanted to sleep. My life revolved around waiting for the FedEx or UPS truck to pull up and deliver my next bottle of Vicodin. When I would run out early, I'd get very sick, and my husband would have to miss work to take care of our son. I hated myself so much, and the guilt and shame I was feeling just made my addiction stronger. I felt alone and so very ashamed.

---

* Name changed to protect privacy

My husband knew I was addicted but didn't know the extent of it. About a year ago, he asked me, and I came clean about it. I also came clean to my therapist as well. They both said they would support me in whatever I needed to do to get clean. I was so ready to be clean. I had tried so many times by myself to taper, but I just wasn't strong enough. So, I went to a detox clinic and started on Suboxone.

The program was for 4 days on Suboxone to help the withdrawal process. A month later, I was back on Vicodin, and I picked up right where I left off. I tried Suboxone again 3 months later, and a few days after I was done with the Sub, I became very ill from something unrelated. I spent a week in the hospital on very heavy pain meds. When I came out of the hospital, they sent me home with a prescription for Vicodin. I spent the next month back on them, and then I went back on Suboxone.

My history proved that the time on Suboxone was just too short. So, I'm now on a maintenance dose of 8 mg of Suboxone, and it's been 3 months since I've taken a Vicodin. The first month I still had bad cravings, but the second month got a little easier, even though I still thought about them. The third month I had no cravings. I feel really good. I'm back to doing all the things I used to do. I don't feel anything from the Suboxone except normal. I can look at myself in the mirror again and feel good about myself. I have my life back. More importantly, my son has his mother back.

- Ashley T Worcester, MA

Now that you have a better idea of the overview of what is involved in MAT, let's take a more in depth look at the process and the medications that are a part of it. This will help when making a decision based on the type of treatment you would like to pursue, especially since MAT is so commonly used.

Let's Stabilize You... Medically Speaking

When you visit a Medication-Assisted Treatment facility, one of the staff's first goals will be to stabilize you medically. It might take a few days, but we will get you there. It is recommended to be off all opiates for 24 to 48 hours prior to starting buprenorphine. On the first day, the medication will start stabilizing the withdrawal symptoms. Within 24 to 48 hours of taking the scheduled doses, cravings and withdrawal should have dropped and stability should begin.

What to Expect at a MAT Facility

Your first visit to a facility will always be the longest. The staff will want to learn about your medical history and your current state of addiction.

When we're asked what a patient should look for in a doctor, we almost always state that the number one quality a doctor should have is empathy. The doctor you're working with should understand the difficulty of actually making the call for an appointment and the even bigger struggle of showing up. A treatment facility should be both empathetic and respectful. One that treats you as an individual without any stigma attached.

At Recovery Connection, one of the things we look for when hiring people is that they have a background or some first-hand experience in dealing with addiction because the staff should have some understanding of where patients are coming from. An empathetic practitioner will want to listen to your story and help you develop a plan for treatment.

Don't Fear the Doctor

One thing that's important to note is that your doctor is your partner. You shouldn't feel like you have to hide any part of your addiction. The more your doctor understands about your addiction and condition, the better they will be able to treat you. The doctor isn't on some kind of pedestal because they've gone to school for countless years and earned a doctorate. Your doctor is a person just like you, and it's important to have a constructive partnership with them. But, before your doctor can truly be your advocate, you must be honest with yourself first. Then, you can be honest with the doctor. This will help you the most.

Your First Visit

It's your first time going in for treatment. You're nervous and you have no idea what to expect. When you arrive, you are greeted by the facility's manager. You will be asked to complete a number of forms. These will help the manager, doctor, and counselor gain a sense of where you are coming from. The forms may touch on questions about your social history, health history, economic history, psychological history, and current medications. You will also be asked to sign a waiver for HIPAA and pharmacy release purposes.

The purpose of your first appointment at a Medication-Assisted Therapy center is to help you get a handle on cravings and withdrawals, but also to approach addiction logically instead of reactively. By getting cravings and other symptoms under control, patients can usually begin to see some light at the end of the tunnel; they can envision a future where they aren't abusing drugs.

Medication for Therapy

The medication part of medication-assisted treatment is designed to do three main things:

- Reduce/prevent detox symptoms

- Make the recovery process as comfortable as possible

- Chemically stabilize opioid receptors

How Effective is Suboxone Therapy?

In virtually all peer-reviewed studies, buprenorphine (the generic term for Suboxone) outperforms placebo. So, Suboxone therapy works (for the most part). But it's not a perfect system.

Dosage

In the early days of Medication-Assisted Therapy that uses buprenorphine, numerous practitioners concluded hastily that they weren't seeing the type of success rates that they should have been seeing. It was later found that many of these practitioners were hesitant to prescribe higher doses of buprenorphine, which limited the effectiveness of treatment early on. Now, the standard treatment amount is up to 8 milligrams on the first day and then 16 milligrams starting on the second day of treatment.

That first dose will help prevent further increase in withdrawal symptoms. The following daily dosages will obtain patient comfort. The reason for the lower dosage on the first day is because we usually ask patients to forego opiates for at least 24 hours before taking the first dose of buprenorphine. That first dose will help curb withdrawal symptoms and the higher dose will help maintain patient comfort.

PATIENT TREATMENT CONTRACT

As a participant in buprenorphine treatment for opioid misuse and dependence, I freely and voluntarily agree to accept this treatment contract as follows:

1. I agree to keep and be on time to all my scheduled appointments.

2. I agree to adhere to the payment policy outlined by this office.

3. I agree to conduct myself in a courteous manner in the doctor's office.

4. I agree no to sell, share, or give any of my medication to another person. I understand that such mishandling of my medication is a serious violation of this agreement and would result in my treatment being terminated without any recourse for appeal.

5. I agree not to deal, steal, or conduct any illegal or disruptive activities in the doctor's office.

6. I understand that if dealing or stealing or if any illegal or disruptive activities are observed or suspected by employees of the pharmacy where my buprenorphine is filled, that the behavior will be reported to my doctor's office and could result in my treatment being terminated without any recourse for appeal.

7. I agree that my medication/prescription can only be given to me at my regular office visits. A missed visit may result in my not being able to get my medication/prescription until the next scheduled visit.

8. I agree that the medication I receive is my responsibility and I agree to keep it in a safe, secure place. I agree that lost medication will not be replaced regardless of why it was lost.

9. I agree not to obtain medications from any doctors, pharmacies, or other sources without telling my treating physician.

10. I understand that mixing buprenorphine with other medications, especially benzodiazepines (for example, Valium®, Klonopin ®, or Xanax ®), can be dangerous. I also recognize that several deaths have occurred among persons mixing buprenorphine and benzodiazepines (especially if taken outside the care of a physician, using routes of administration other than sublingual or in higher than recommended therapeutic doses).

11. I agree to take my medication as my doctor has instructed and not to alter the way I take my medication without first consulting my doctor.

12. I understand that medication alone is not sufficient treatment for my condition, and I agree to participate in counseling as discussed and agreed upon with my doctor and specified in my treatment plan.

13. I agree to abstain from alcohol, opioids, marijuana, cocaine, and other addictive substances (excepting nicotine).

14. I agree to provide random urine samples and have my doctor test my blood alcohol level.

15. I understand that violations of the above may be grounds for termination of treatment.

_____   _____

Patient Signature   Date

_____   _____

Physician Signature   Date

EXPLANATION OF TREATMENT

Intake

You will be given a comprehensive substance dependence assessment, as well as an evaluation of mental status and physical exam. The pros and cons of the medication, SUBOXONE, will be presented. Treatment expectations, as well as issues involved with maintenance versus medially supervised withdrawal will be discussed.

Induction

You will be switched from you current opioid (heroin, methadone, or prescription painkillers) on to SUBOXONE. At the time of induction, you will be asked to provide a urine sample to confirm the presence of opioids and possible other drugs. You must arrive for the first visit experience mild to moderate opioid withdrawal symptoms. Arrangements will be made for you to receive your first dose shortly after your initial appointment. Your response to the initial dose will be monitored. You may receive additional medication, if necessary, to reduce your withdrawal symptoms.

Since an individual's tolerance and reaction to SUBOXONE vary, daily appointments may be scheduled and medications will be adjusted until you no longer experience withdrawal symptoms or cravings. Urine drug screening is typically required for all patients at every visit during this phase.

Intake and Induction may both occur at the first visit, depending on your needs and your doctor's evaluation.

Stabilization

Once the appropriate dose of SUBOXONE is established, you will stay at this dose until steady blood levels are achieved. You and your doctor will discuss your treatment options form this point forward.

Maintenance

Treatment compliance and progress with be monitored. Participation in some form of behavioral counseling is strongly recommended to ensure best chance of treatment success. You are likely to have scheduled appointments on a weekly basis, however, if treatment progress is good and goals are met, monthly visits will eventually be considered sufficient. The Maintenance phase canals from weeks to years-the length of treatment will be determined by you and your doctor, and, possibly, your counselor. Your length of treatment may vary depending on your individual needs.

Medically Supervised Withdrawal

As your treatment progresses, you and your doctor may eventually decide that medically supervised withdrawal is an appropriate option for you. In this phase, your doctor will gradually taper your SUBOXONE dose over time, taking care to see that you do not experience any withdrawal symptoms or cravings.

EXPLANATION OF 1ST VISIT—No In-Office Supply

Your first visit is generally the longest, and may last anywhere from 1 to 4 hours.

Before you can be seen by the doctor, all of your paperwork must be completed. In order to set up your initial visit with the doctor, all paperwork must completely filled out and received by our office. In addition, you will need to pay the doctor's fees prior to the start of treatment.

When preparing for your 1st office visit, there are a couple of logistical issues you may want to consider.

- You may not want to return to work after your visit-this is very normal, so just plan accordingly.

- Because SUBOXONE can cause drowsiness and slow reaction times, particularly during the 1st few weeks of treatment, driving yourself home after the 1st visit is generally not recommended, so you may want to make arrangements for a ride home.

  It is very important to arrive for your 1st visit already experiencing mild to moderate opioid withdrawal symptoms. If you are in withdrawal, buprenorphine will help lessen the symptoms. However, if you are not in withdrawal, buprenorphine will "override" the opioids already in your system, which will cause severe withdrawal symptoms.

The following guidelines are provided to ensure you are in withdrawal for the visit. (If this concerns you, it may help to schedule your first visit in the morning: some patients find it easiest to skip what would normally be their first dose of the day).

- No methadone or long-acting painkillers for at least 24 hours.

- No heroin or short-acting painkillers for at least 4 to 6 hours.

Bring ALL medication bottles with you to your 1st appointment.

Urine drug screening is a regular feature of SUBOXONE therapy, because it provides physicians with important insights into your health and your treatment. Your 1st visit will include urine drug screening, and may also entail a Breathalyzer ® test and blood work. If you haven't had a recent physical exam, your doctor may require one. To help ensure that SUBOXONE is the best treatment option for you, your doctor will perform a substance dependence assessment and mental status evaluation. Lastly, you and your doctor will discuss SUBOXONE and your expectations of treatment.

After this portion of your visit is completed, your doctor will most likely give you a SUBOXONE prescription. A prescription cannot be guaranteed prior to your visit with the doctor. You fill the prescription at the pharmacy and return to the doctor's office so you can take the medication in a safe place where the medical staff can monitor your response.

Your response to the medication will be evaluated after 1 hour and possibly again after 2 hours. Once the doctor is comfortable with your response, you can schedule your next visit and go home. Your doctor may ask you to keep a record of any medications you take at home to control withdrawal symptoms. You will also receive instructions on how to contact your doctor in emergency, as well as additional information about treatment.

CHECKLIST FOR 1st VISIT:

- **Fees prepaid** prior to first visit (cash, check or credit card)
- Paperwork received prior to first visit
- Arrive experiencing mild to moderate **opioid withdrawal** symptoms
- Arrive with a **full bladder**
- Bring **ALL medication bottles**

Starting Suboxone: A Patient's Guide

You can't just start or stop using Suboxone—you have to be eased onto and off of it. The process of easing you onto Suboxone is called induction.

Before Induction: Heroin, prescription painkillers, and methadone all belong to a family of drugs called the opioids. Before you start on Suboxone, your doctor will ask you to stay off all opioids for a little while—usually less than a day. The exact amount of time you'll need to stay off opioids depends on what kind of drugs you've been taking and how much you use per day.

After going for a day or two without using opioids, you will be in the early stages of withdrawal. You may feel uncomfortable for a little while, but you will feel better when you start taking Suboxone.

If you do slip up and use an opioid during this time, you run the risk of going into sudden, intense withdrawal. Tell your doctor if you used opiods, and he or she will reschedule your induction.

During induction: Over the course of a few days (usually 1-3 days), your physician will gradually increase your dose of Suboxone until he or she finds your ideal dose. During this time:

Don't use any opiods—you will probably go into withdrawal and be very uncomfortable! Do expect to spend and extended period of time in the doctor's office—your doctor may need to keep you under observation while you adjust to the medication.

Do be prepared for a few days of craving—you may crave opiods until the Suboxone begins to kick in, but it is very important that you do not use them!

Do be honest with your physician how you're feeling—your doctor needs to know about your mood, your level of craving, and your physical state to accurately determine your ideal dose of Suboxone.

After Induction:

Don't stop using Suboxone without talking to your doctor—you will go into withdrawal. Do tell you doctor if you experience side effects due to the Suboxone or if you crave opioids— your dose may need to be adjusted if you do.

Do take advantage of therapy and other resources that can help you stay drug free and stable! Buprenorphine/Naloxone Combination Tablets—What do they mean for You?

Your physician has prescribed buprenorphine/naloxone combination tablets for you. There are a few things you should know about this tablet before you begin taking it.

What is buprenorphine?

Buprenorphine is a type of drug called an opioid, similar to heroin, methadone or oxycontin. Taking buprenorphine will prevent you from going into withdrawal and should stop you from craving other opioids.

What is naloxone?

Naloxone counteracts opiods—including buprenorphine. If you take naloxone while you have an opioid in your system, or if you are dependent on opioids and find that you go into withdrawal without them, naloxone can trigger withdrawal.

That doesn't make sense—why would my doctor prescribe a drug which will send me into withdrawal?

Your buprenorphine/naloxone combination tablets will not send you into withdrawal—provided you take time as your doctor prescribes.

If you dissolve the tablets under your tongue, or if you accidentally swallow one, the naloxone will not affect you—your body breaks the naloxone down too quickly for it to take effect.

However, if you inject a combination tablet, the naloxone will take effect. You will probably not feel anything from the buprenorphine, and you could go into withdrawal.

So-always take you Suboxone as your physician prescribes it. Don't inject it, and don't allow others to inject it.

How Taken	Buprenorphine	Naloxone	What you feel
Under the tongue (as directed)	Works properly	Broken down by the body	No withdrawal; reduced craving
Swallowed (accidental)	Broken down by the body	Broken down by the body	Medicine will not work; you could go into withdrawal or feel cravings
Injected (abuse)	Blocked by naloxone	Blocks effect of opioids	You could go into withdrawal very quickly

Keys to Successful Addiction Treatment

Overcoming an addiction is not easy—it takes courage and commitment. However, as many people have discovered, the rewards of going clean and staying sober are worth the effort.

Starting treatment is an important first step toward overcoming drug use. If you follow the guidelines listed below, your treatment will be much more effective, and you will have a better chance of staying drug-free. These keys to successful treatment are based on medical research and the experiences of thousands of patients who successfully stopped using drugs during treatment and remained drug-free afterwards.

✂ Above all else, stay in treatment. Patients who stay in treatment have a much better chance of staying drug-free than those who drop out.

✂ Especially for the first month of treatment, you may feel very unmotivated to continue. This is normal—most patients who drop out of treatment do so in the first 30 days. You need to be prepared for this feeling so you can better resist the urge to drop out.

✂ Obey the program's rules—they're in place to help you become drug-free. Also, many programs will stop your treatment if you don't follow the rules.

✂ Develop a good relationship with your doctor or counselor. Many people who have gone on to become drug-free have found that trusting relationships with their counselors were important in helping them complete treatment.

✂ Make a commitment to your treatment and to changing you life. Don't just go to all your treatment sessions-take part in them too.

✂ Follow your treatment plan and use the services that your doctor or counselor recommends.

✂ Don't let a lapse become a relapse. Many people lapse and use drugs once, twice, or even more times during treatment. If this happens to you, it doesn't mean that your treatment has failed— but it does mean that you're having trouble. Talk to you doctor or counselor about the lapse, and let them help you stop it from becoming a relapse-a return to drug abuse.

✂ Ask for help if you need it! That's what you doctor of counselor is there for.

✕ Be prepared to make some major life changes. It's very hard to stay sober when the people around you are still using drugs. You will need to stay away from friends who use drugs and, if possible, get out of houses or even neighborhoods where drug use is going on.

Follow these keys to treatment and you will be on your way to a drug-free life!

Common Side Effects of Suboxone

Suboxone is safe to use for most patients. Some people do experience side effects, but most of Suboxone's side effects are not dangerous—they're just unpleasant.

Common minor side effects include:

- Nausea
- Sweating
- Constipation
- Headache
- Drowsiness
- Depression
- Disturbed Sleep

If you experience any of the above, talk to your doctor. Your doctor may give you medicine to treat the side effects, or your doctor may lower your dose of Suboxone slightly. Regardless, most minor side effects will either go away as you become used to the drug or can be treated with minor lifestyle changes.

Some people with certain medical conditions are at risk for more serious side effects:

Drug Interactions: Some people who take both sedatives and Suboxone have overdosed on one or both drugs. If you have been prescribed medications, make certain your doctor knows. He or she may change how much of each drug you take. Also, while on Suboxone never take sedatives r other drugs except those prescribed by your doctor!

Allergic Reaction: If you develop hives or a rash while taking Suboxone, you may be allergic to it. If this happens, call your doctor or go to the emergency room immediately. Also, tell your doctor if you know that you are allergic to drugs called buprenorphine or naloxone.

Respiratory Depression: Like prescription narcotics and heroin, Suboxone affects the reflexes that keep you breathing. In most patients, this effect is minimal, but it can be serious in patients who already have damaged or diseased lungs. If you have a condition that impairs your breathing, tell your doctor before beginning Suboxone.

Liver Problems (hepatitis): A few people have developed problems with their livers while taking Suboxone. Most of these people already had liver problems like hepatitis B or C or cirrhosis due to alcohol abuse. If you have had liver problems in the past, make sure that your doctor knows. He or she will monitor you liver closely during your treatment. If you develop severe stomach pain, severe nausea, or jaundice (skin and/or whites of the eyes look yellow), get to the hospital as quickly as possible. Your chances of full recovery are very good if you get treatment quickly.

Head Injury: If you have suffered a severe head injury or have been told by a doctor that you have an intracranial lesion, tell your doctor before beginning Suboxone. Suboxone causes an increase in pressure in the skull, and this can make your injury worse.

FREQUENTLY ASKED QUESTIONS-PATIENTS

1. **Why do I have to feel sick to start the medication for it to work best?**

   When you take your first dose of Suboxone, if you already have high levels of another opioid in your system, the Suboxone will compete with those opioid molecules and replace them at the receptor sites. Because Suboxone has milder opioid effects than full agonist opioid, you may go into a rapid opioid

   Withdrawal and feel sick, a condition which is called "precipitated withdrawal."

   By already being in mild to moderate withdrawal when you take your first dose of Suboxone, the medication will make you feel noticeably better, not worse.

2. **How does Suboxone work?**

   Suboxone binds to the same receptors as other opioid drugs. It mimics the effects of other opioids by alleviating cravings and withdrawal symptoms. This allows you to address the psychosocial reasons behind your opioid use.

3. **When will I start to feel better?**

   Most patients feel a measurable improvement by 30 minutes, with the full effects clearly noticeable after about 1 hour.

4. **How long will Suboxone last?**

   After the first hour, many people say they feel pretty good for most of the day. Responses to Suboxone will vary based on factors such as tolerance and metabolism, so each patient's dosing is individualized. Your doctor may increase your dose of Suboxone during the first week to help keep you from feeling sick.

5. **Can I go to work right after my first dose?**

Suboxone can cause drowsiness and slow reaction times. These responses are more likely over the first few weeks of treatment, when your dose is being adjusted. During this time, your ability to drive, operate machinery, and play sports may be affected. Some people do go to work right after their first Suboxone dose, however, many people prefer to take the first and possibly the second day off until they feel better.

If you are concerned about missing work, talk with your physician about possible ways to minimize the possibility of your taking time off (e.g. Scheduling your induction on a Friday).

6. **Is it important to take my medication at the same time each day?**

In order to make sure that you do not get sick, it is important to take your medication at the same time every day.

7. **If I have more than one tablet, do I need to take them together at the same time?**

Yes and no- you do need to take your dose at one "sitting," but you do not necessarily need to fit all the tablets under your tongue simultaneously. Some people prefer to take their tablets this way because it's faster, but this may not be what works best for you. The most important thing is to be sure to take the full daily dose you were prescribed, so that your body maintains constant levels of Suboxone.

8. **Why does Suboxone need to be placed under the tongue?**

There are two large veins under your tongue (you can see them with a mirror). Placing the medication under your tongue allows Suboxone to be absorbed quickly and safely through these veins as the tablet dissolves. If you chew of swallow your medication, it will not be correctly absorbed as it is extensively metabolized by the liver. Similarly, if the medication is not allowed to dissolve completely, you won't receive the full effect.

9. **Why can't I talk while the medication is dissolving under my tongue?**

When you talk, you move your tongue, which lets the undissolved Suboxone "leak" out from underneath, thereby preventing it from being absorbed by the two veins. Entertaining yourself by reading or watching television while your medication dissolves can help the time to pass more quickly.

10. **Why does it sometimes only take 5 minutes for Suboxone to dissolve and other times it takes much longer?**

Generally, it takes about 5-10 minutes for a tablet to dissolve. However, other factors (e.g. the moisture of your mouth) can effect that time. Drinking something before taking your medication is a good way to help the tablet dissolve more quickly.

11. **If I forget to take my Suboxone for a day will I feel sick?**

Suboxone works best when taken every 24 hours, however, it may last longer than 24 hours, so you may not get sick. If you miss your dose, try to take it as soon as possible, unless it is almost time for your next dose. If it is almost time for your next dose, just skip the dose you forgot, and take next dose as prescribed. Do not take two doses at once unless directed to do so by your physician.

In the future, the best way to help yourself remember to take your medication is to start taking it at the same time that you perform a routine, daily activity, such as when you get dressed in the morning. This way, the daily activity will start to serve as a reminder to take your Suboxone.

12. What happens if I still feel sick after taking Suboxone for a while?

There are some reasons why you may still feel sick. You may not be taking the medication correctly or the dose may not be right for you. It is important to tell your doctor or nurse if you still feel sick.

13. What happens if I take drugs and then take Suboxone?

You will probably feel very sick and experience what is called a "precipitated withdrawal." Suboxone competes with other opioids and will displace those opioid molecules from the receptors. Because Suboxone has less opioid effects than full agonist opioids, you will go into withdrawal and feel sick.

14. What happens if I take Suboxone and then take drugs?

As long as Suboxone is in your body, it will significantly reduce the effects of any other opioids used, because Suboxone will dominate the receptor sites and block other opioids from producing any effect.

15. What are the side effects of this medication?

Some of the most common side effects that patients experience are nausea, headache, constipation, and body aches and pains. However, most side effects seen with Suboxone appear during the first week or two of treatment, and then generally subside. If you are experiencing any side effects, be sure to talk about it with your doctor or nurse, as s/he can often treat those symptoms effectively until they abate on their own.

Understanding Opioid Dependence

Opioid dependence is a disease in which there are biological or physical, psychological, and social changes. Some of the physical changes include the need for increasing amounts of opioid to produce the same effect, symptoms of withdrawal, feeling of craving and changes in sleep patterns. Psychological components of opioid dependence include a reliance on heroin or other drugs to help you cope with everyday problems or inability to feel good or celebrate without using heroin or opioids. The social components of opioid dependence include less frequent contact with important people in your life, and an inability to participate in important events due to drug use. In extreme cases, there may even be criminal and legal implications.

The hallmarks of opioid dependence are the continued use of drugs despite their negative effect, the need for increasing amounts of opioids to have the same effect and the development of withdrawal symptoms upon cessation.

There are a variety of factors that can contribute to the continued use of opioids. Among these are the use of heroin to escape from or cope with problems, the need to use increasing amounts of heroin to achieve the same effect, and the need for a "high."

Treatment

Treatment for opioid dependence is best considered a long-term process.

Recovery from opioid dependence is not an easy or painless process, as it involves changes in drug use and lifestyle, such as adopting new coping skills. Recovery can involve hard work, commitment, discipline, and a willingness to examine the effects of opioid dependence on your life. At first, it isn't unusual to feel impatient, angry, or frustrated.

The changes you need to make will depend on how opioid dependence has specifically affected your life. The following are some of the common areas of change to think about when developing your specific recovery plan:

Physical-good nutrition, exercise, sleep and relaxation.

Emotional-learning to cope with feelings, problems, stresses and negative thinking without relying on opioids.

Social-developing relationships with sober people, learning to resist pressures from others to use or misuse substances, and developing healthy social and leisure interest to occupy your time and give you a sense of satisfactions and pleasure.

Family-examining the impact opioid dependence has had on your family, encouraging them to get involved in your treatment, mending relationships with family members, and working hard to have mutually satisfying relationships with family members.

Spiritual-learning to listen to your inner voice for support and strength, and using that voice to guide you in developing a renewed sense of purpose and meaning.

During the treatment process, Suboxone will help you avoid many or all of the physical symptoms of opioid withdrawal. These typically include craving, restlessness, poor sleep, irritability, yawning, muscle cramps, runny nose, tearing, goose-flesh, nausea, vomiting and diarrhea. Your doctor may prescribe other medications for you as necessary to help relieve these symptoms.

You should be careful not to respond to these withdrawal symptoms by losing patience with the treatment process and thinking that the symptoms can only be corrected by using drugs. To help you deal with the symptoms of withdrawal, you should try to set small goals and work towards them.

Environment

The environment that supports treatment matters, which is also evidenced by the disparate success rates of comparative studies. Environmental factors which can influence the effectiveness of treatment can include not only the design of the treatment program and staff, but also the physical location. Additionally, the proximity of the treatment center to public transportation routes can affect participation rates among those without reliable transportation.

The Human Factor

The biggest factor influencing how successful your treatment will be is your determination. Yes, buprenorphine will decrease withdrawals, cravings and the urge to use. However, your utilization of counseling to learn safe and proper behaviors is key to your success. Recovery is learning the tools to make better decisions and doing them.

There's also the factor of taking the medication correctly. Some forms of buprenorphine must be taken under the tongue, and you might have to keep it there for 10 minutes or more for it to be properly absorbed. Some patients have the mistaken belief that swallowing the tablet has the same effect, but it is absorbed differently. Therefore, this could lead some patients to believe that the medication isn't as effective as it should be.

The effectiveness of Medication-Assisted Therapies has helped to curb the perceived stigmatization of using medications in the treatment of opioid use disorders. In addition to medication, Medication-Assisted Treatments also combine behavioral therapies and counseling to help patients stay on track to recovery.

What About Methadone?

If you enter a methadone treatment program, you can expect that for roughly a year (on average), you will be receiving an oral methadone dose each morning. Usually, these centers are open from 5 AM to 9 AM. When you go there, you will usually be given a dose between 60 and 120 milligrams or more. Once you've done that for the better part of a year and your drug screens are going well, they will usually allow you to start taking methadone doses at home.

For the longest time, methadone treatment centers were the only option when it came to treating opiate-dependent patients. Most patients who undergo methadone therapy are referred by a physician. However, there are most likely methadone treatment centers in your area that accept walk-in patients. In our state of Rhode Island, CODAC, would be one such facility where you do not need a referral to start receiving treatments.

Now, you're probably wondering if there's a better outpatient option other than methadone clinics. The answer is yes.

Buprenorphine

Buprenorphine is a prescription drug that is used as a replacement to heroin, morphine, and methadone dependence. When one prescription drug is used to replace an illicit drug, this is known as pharmacotherapy. Buprenorphine starts off with weekly visits to a buprenorphine provider. So, unlike methadone, you will only need to start buprenorphine treatment by going once a week. During these weekly visits, you are not only receiving your buprenorphine doses for the week, but you are also connecting with doctors and counselors that will work with you in developing a treatment plan.

When we discuss Suboxone therapy, we are trying to speak in simpler terms since Suboxone is actually the most well-known brand name of buprenorphine. And, we have to admit that it's way easier to spell and say Suboxone, compared to buprenorphine.

Making the Choice: Methadone or Buprenorphine (Suboxone or Sublocade)

In terms of Medication-Assisted Treatments for those looking to win the fight against opioids, you essentially have two choices: methadone or buprenorphine.

One of the biggest questions when it comes to Medication-Assisted Therapies is which one to try first.

Suboxone (buprenorphine) and methadone are the two most popular options for those seeking MAT. Each type of treatment has its own pros and cons, so in this section we will break down the pros and cons to give you a better grasp of which type of treatment might work best for you.

Methadone

Methadone is a synthetic opiate that binds to certain receptors in the brain, which helps to stabilize the body for a period of time. It's not a full opiate. It can be a risk or a threat to take as well, if someone overdoses on it or abuses it. Methadone was the beginning of medication-assisted treatment. Even though buprenorphine is available, there is still a place in the treatment spectrum for methadone. Methadone has been available since the 1950s and 1960s. It served an important purpose in helping those with opiate dependency to safely ween off illicit substances.

Even though methadone treatment has been around for nearly 70 years, there's a reason that people still choose methadone over the newer options. The major reason is that methadone treatment is a day-to-day process. You develop a routine of going to the methadone clinic each morning for that day's dose. There's also that built-in risk of losing the treatment option; some methadone facilities may refuse to treat a patient if they miss a day. Plus, there is a very real possibility that you could go into withdrawals if you do miss treatment after consecutive days.

The people that do the best in methadone treatment are those that prefer a daily, regimented program. But there is also a specific group who may prefer methadone, which is pregnant women. Opiate-dependent women who become pregnant are usually recommended to methadone treatment. Another group that can benefit from methadone treatment is patients who have not achieved success with other programs and have gone through multiple hospitalizations or detoxes. Methadone treatment may allow these individuals to get a better grasp on treatment and follow through with the program.

The reason that methadone clinics are so thorough in making you sure you take the treatment (and they do check) is that methadone can be abused by taking more than the prescribed amount. That is why most clinics won't allow patients to take home a multi-day supply of methadone because it can be abused.

In cases where a person is a recovering heroin user and maybe they are part of a court-mandated treatment program, they may prefer methadone since it does provide a good amount of relief in a way similar to heroin. But methadone treatment can be lengthy. When you go through treatment, you usually increase by 10 milligram increments until you reach an ideal maintenance level. But the clinics then slowly withdrawal patients at one milligram a week. You could start off at 60, 70, or even over a hundred milligrams a week, so you can see that the winding down process can take quite a lot of time. But, if it works, it works.

The philosophy of why most methadone treatment centers will start you out on a high dose is that they want you to feel good and stable during that first phase of recovery, so therefore they are willing to overshoot, if that's what it takes. You might have a little "buzz" taking the morning dose of methadone, but the goal is to make sure you are a productive and responsible member of society. The withdrawal period is long because the main goal isn't just to get you off opioids but to get you off opioids gently.

Cons of methadone

The downside of methadone treatment is that it takes years, not months, to come off of methadone. One other side effect of methadone is that — like opiates — it can make you somewhat drowsy during the afternoon, usually between 4 PM to 6 PM. This is known as the "sundown" phase.

There have been some methadone patients who have been forced to come off methadone due to failing numerous urine screens. Some patients describe methadone withdrawal as feeling like you've been hit by a train or that an earthquake has happened internally and it's shaking your bones. There's also the feeling of excruciating pain throughout your body. The pain of going through methadone withdrawal can be too much for some and they will search out any form of relief, even if that means seeking out heroin or another opiate.

Suboxone/Buprenorphine

Buprenorphine is another tool in the tool chest of fighting addiction. Buprenorphine is the chemical drug name for Suboxone. The two are entirely identical. But due to the hard-to-pronounce (and hard to spell) nature of buprenorphine, most people refer to it as simply Suboxone. This is similar in a way to how people, when asking for a facial tissue, ask for a Kleenex, even though Kleenex is just a brand of facial tissue.

What is Suboxone?

Suboxone is a combination of buprenorphine and naloxone. Naloxone is a derivative similar to Narcan, which is compounded with naloxone in order to make the drug less susceptible to diversion.

Buprenorphine is a partial opiate. Most drug users, especially those coming from injecting, will know that the way to get a fast, intense high is to inject the drug. But, when buprenorphine and naloxone are injected together, you are essentially also injecting yourself with Narcan.

When buprenorphine is taken the correct way (as a dissolvable in the mouth), very little of the Naloxone is absorbed through the mucosa (the lining of the mouth). But much of the buprenorphine is absorbed and will cover the opioid receptors.

So that's the primary reason naloxone is added to buprenorphine, to discourage diversion. If you do try to inject it, any sort of high will be canceled out by the naloxone since you would essentially be injecting a partial opiate and naloxone. This essentially places someone in immediate [florid] withdrawal. Of course, immediate withdrawal can also make you feel very sick.

How Do They Know if I Took the Buprenorphine?

When you visit the clinic for buprenorphine, they should always make you take a urine screen. What they are looking for is metabolites of buprenorphine to make sure that you are actually taking the medication.

There have actually been some individuals who think they are going to beat the system by just placing suboxone film into their urine screen but doing this will actually be apparent during a urine screen since it will just show the drug, not the metabolite. In the readout, buprenorphine metabolites show up as [NOR buprenorphine], indicating that it is the metabolite of the drug.

What is Suboxone Film?

When Suboxone first came out, it was in the form of a tablet. Around 2010, the film variety of Suboxone came out. This is a type of dissolvable film that is similar to Listerine tabs. These films are designed to dissolve faster under the tongue. This is seen as a more comfortable option for patients since the drug dissolves quickly and there isn't all the foamy spit like with the tablets.

Taking Suboxone Film Correctly

Suboxone film is placed under the tongue and absorbed through the mucosa. If it's swallowed or you take a drink or smoke during that 7-to-10-minute duration, then less of the drug is likely to be absorbed into your blood stream. So, it's important to not swallow or drink anything during those 7 to 10 minutes when the buprenorphine strip is dissolving under the tongue.

Recently Suboxone stopped being reimbursed by a lot of insurance companies because the patent expired. Now, there are several generic companies manufacturing the genericized version of the tablet. It is also likely that there will be a generic form of the Suboxone film.

To be considered a generic, the drug has to be at least 80% chemically identical to the original. For this reason, some patients may not have the same sort of response to the generic as they did with name-brand Suboxone. You could also encounter differences with the taste where one patient will prefer one over the other. This may not make a difference treatment-wise, but it does matter to some patients. A medically necessary brand can be requested if these symptoms have been established/occur.

Tablets vs. Film

In the end, everything comes down to how effective the treatment is, and that means that there should be little difference between Suboxone tablets and the film so long as the dose is taken correctly. Since the film version dissolves quicker, it is usually more fool proof in terms of getting the right dose. Dissolvable tablets, on the other hand, take a little longer to dissolve, which means the duration can be affected by the amount of saliva in the mouth and even the chemistry of the individual patient's saliva.

"I tried Suboxone from a friend but didn't like it." We've heard this statement several times from people after their first try of Suboxone from a friend or acquaintance that led to a negative reaction because it made them sick. Unfortunately, this leads many people who would otherwise benefit from buprenorphine being turned off from the treatment because they simply did not take it the correct way.

Pros of Buprenorphine

There are a number of positive aspects of buprenorphine treatment. For one, buprenorphine is considered the "gold standard" of treatment for those addicted to opiates. One of the major benefits of choosing treatment with buprenorphine is that you will be doing something good for yourself. You are virtually eliminating the possibility of overdosing or getting some substance that may be laced with fentanyl. One of the things that many patients find relieving about buprenorphine treatment is that it is essentially as discrete as you want it to be. You are not waiting outside a methadone clinic each morning and you can take the medication in the privacy of your own home.

Cons of Buprenorphine

One of the main cons of buprenorphine is that you are still taking a medication that is a partial opiate, so there may be some stigmatization there. You may have people telling you that you have a crutch.

The other downside of buprenorphine is that it's still an opiate. So, if you miss a dose or two, you will begin to feel some degree of withdrawal. Because buprenorphine has an extended half-life, you will likely not begin to experience withdrawals for several days. When you suddenly stop taking the medication (not titrating), the symptoms of withdrawal can be unpleasant. So, if you miss a day of medication, you should not begin withdrawal symptoms until the following day. Further, if you fail to take your medication for a longer period of time, withdrawal symptoms will increase.

Methadone Centers Offering Buprenorphine Treatment

With the realization that treating drug dependency isn't a one-size-fits-all solution, many methadone treatment centers are now offering buprenorphine treatments. Some of this has to do with perceived regulatory hurdles (many were under the mistaken belief that in order to switch over to buprenorphine-based Medication-Assisted Treatments they would need to shut down the methadone side of their operation). But there is also an issue of funding. Many methadone clinics are funded by government programs; therefore, they were hesitant to change.

Zubsolv v. Suboxone

Zubsolv is another brand of buprenorphine-based treatment that is out there. Whether you are prescribed Zubsolv, Suboxone, or a generic brand will largely come down to the preferences of your insurance company. But, by and large, Zubsolv and Suboxone essentially have the same proportion of buprenorphine and naloxone.

It's important to note that if you frequently go to different pharmacies to have your prescription filled, since buprenorphine is a controlled substance, it's very easy to trigger a warning at the pharmacy. This can happen if you are filling prescriptions at two, three, or more pharmacies. You might be doing nothing wrong, but to the inter-pharmacy system, it looks suspicious when you have prescriptions filled at different pharmacies. To avoid this pitfall (and possibly a lapse in treatment), it's best to stick to one or two local pharmacies.

What is Subutex?

Subutex is pure buprenorphine without the abuse-dissuading naloxone. Since this drug can be abused, it is typically only available to patients that have had an adverse reaction to the naloxone, such as a severe allergy. Currently, the parent company that manufactured Subutex is no longer manufacturing this medication, but it is still being made in its generic form.

You should know that many doctors are aware that people are looking to abuse pure buprenorphine, so if you are wanting to get a script with pure buprenorphine you will actually need to demonstrate that you are really allergic to the naloxone. Beyond allergies, Subutex is used for patients who are pregnant, since naloxone can cause pregnancy complications. Also, a naloxone allergy is quite rare.

What is Sublocade?

Sublocade is buprenorphine in an injectable form. The great thing about this form of treatment is that the drug is delivered as a once-a-month injectable. Therefore, it's a long-lasting form of treatment. After an injection, you could potentially go 45 days until you begin symptoms of withdrawal. Compare that to Suboxone, where you could go into withdrawal in as little as three to five days (if you fail to take your doses), and Sublocade could be a better option for you. The first 2 doses are called loading doses. The first and second month is 300 mg, and then starting the third month, 100 mg maintains the medication level in the body. If a person does not feel supported enough, they can go back to 300 mg monthly. This may seem like a severe drop-off, but you have to consider that the half-life of Sublocade ranges from 40 to 60 days. Therefore, that first dose is still working when you receive your second dose. Sublocade is a subcutaneous injection, meaning it is injected below the skin, not into a vein or muscle.

How does Sublocade last so long?

When Sublocade is injected under the surface of your skin, it forms a sort of gel called atrigel. Essentially, Sublocade becomes a sort of gel which slowly releases a buprenorphine-based chemical. Michael Brier, the CEO of Recovery Connection, has quipped that this is a "storing extra for the winter type of thing." Keeping the level at 2 nanograms will provide you with the biggest blockade and decrease craving and urges.

Ideal Patients for Sublocade

Sublocade provides a sense of decision-making stability. When patients know that their monthly shot will likely interfere with any type of additional pill or injection, they are less likely to make that kind of decision. There are also those "turnstile" or "carousel" patients who are constantly in and out of recovery because they get tripped up, and then they are back to using. Therefore, Sublocade is ideal for individuals who truly want to succeed but they sometimes stumble. It can help prevent them from themselves.

There are some people who just like the convenience of Sublocade and those who would rather not have buprenorphine tablets or film strips in the house. The downside of this, of course, is that the convenience comes by way of a needle, which no one is really a fan of. Sublocade is also ideal for people who have hectic schedules, or they travel extensively. Sublocade has a half-life of 40 to 60 days, which creates a flatter slope to come down on, especially on the last dose. It also means that the therapeutic window will be the same each month.

Depending on the number of months you have been on the injection will determine the amount of time that your therapeutic levels will dip down. If you have taken at least 4 months of injections, you may have 2 months of therapeutic levels within you before experiencing withdrawal symptoms. You then can return back to oral buprenorphine for stabilization.

Here's an important tip: most clinics that offer Sublocade call it into a specialty pharmacy and then it is sent to the clinic. If the clinic doesn't have your correct contact information (especially your phone number), it can cause issues in terms of getting the injection to you on a timely basis.

What Happens if I Inject Heroin or Abuse Other Opiates While on Sublocade?

There was a study conducted with individuals who were administered Sublocade. They were given 18 milligrams of hydromorphone or Dilaudid. They asked patients if there was any effect after the injection. A majority of the patients stated there was no pleasurable effect. This allowed the company making Sublocade to say that it has an opiate-blocking effect up to 18 milligrams. Is it possible to take an amount of 18 milligrams and overdose? Yes, in theory, it is still possible. Therefore, if you somehow slip while on Sublocade, there is enough opioid receptor-blocking action that the effect will be fairly minimal. Therefore, simple slips may not work or create any sort of euphoric effect.

Using Sublocade

Although the Sublocade injection is delivered on a monthly basis, your counselor will still want to see you actively. The frequency of your visits will all depend on where you are coming from in terms of previous drug use and the progression of your treatment. Therefore, your visits with the counselor may be anywhere from twice a week to every two weeks.

So far, the biggest complaint about Sublocades is from the psychological perspective of not taking medication every day. Since it is only taken once a month, some patients may wonder whether the injection is actually working that whole time. When some people take a tablet or dissolvable film each day, they feel like they have achieved a comfort level that they've done what they were supposed to do for the day. So, for some patients, the worry is how effective can a medication be if it is only taken once a month. Your mind can begin to play tricks on you as to whether the medication is actually working. This can lead to psychological cravings that are not actual cravings.

There is also a sort of social safety net when it comes to Sublocade. A person could be around users who could be pressuring them to use. But if they can explain that taking an illicit substance won't do anything for them, then it is an easy situation to get out of. In contrast, if a person is taking a daily dose of buprenorhpine, they could simply say to themselves, "Hey, I can just not take my Suboxone for a few days and go out and have a fun weekend." With a monthly injection, the likelihood of talking yourself into trouble is greatly reduced. This is also where the counseling aspect of treatment comes into play.

Vivitrol: The Most Common Injectable

Vivitrol is an opiate blocker that is injected into the gluteus maximus. For those that are not familiar with human biology, the gluteus maximus is the muscle in your butt. Vivitrol was not originally developed as an opioid treatment but has been adopted by many providers in treating opioid use disorders. Vivitrol is also used in treating alcohol addiction, but if you are truly fighting opioid addiction, Sublocade will most likely be the best option for you.

Length of MAT

Once you've chosen the MAT that works best for you, the question usually arises concerning the time frame. How long will an individual need to stay on their chosen medication. That's usually one of the first questions patients will ask when they start on Suboxone/buprenorphine or Sublocade therapy. One general rule of thumb, and this can change from patient to patient, is to take the number of years of drug use, then multiply that either two or three-fold. This should give you a rough figure of treatment duration. So, it's going to take a while.

Chapter 9
Recovery and Relapse

Dawn's Story*

*My name is Dawn, and I'm 31. I started using OxyContin when I was 15. My older sister gave them to me for cramps, so in my mind, that made it okay to use. I knew that the first time I used, this was **my** drug. It felt like a warm blanket over me. I was a great kid, but after 4 days, I had used all of my sister's pain pills, filled the empty capsules with powdered sugar, and put them back in the bottle so that she wouldn't notice they were all gone. I felt so clever and calm.*

For about 10 years I used one to two times a week. Then in 2009, my dad died so I increased to using every day. Then in 2013, my boyfriend's dad died after being on life support for over a month. During that time, I started using 30 to 40 hydrocodone a day.

I was a full-blown addict. I would try to stop using but would get so sick. I felt powerless. I got up to 50 (10 hydrocodone/325 Tylenol) pills a day. I wasn't getting that good feeling anymore. My family thought that I slurred my words, threw up, and slept all of the time because of my Crohn's Disease. My depression was overwhelming. My doctor kept increasing my anti-depressants. I was hopeless, and I couldn't keep this big, horrible secret anymore. But I tried. I pawned cherished and stolen things. I stole money from loved ones, and I conned people into giving me money. I lost my job of 10 years due to using (but I said that it

---

* Name changed to protect privacy

was because of my Crohn's Disease that I didn't show up to work. And when I did show up, I would leave after a couple of hours).

I lived to use and used to live. I sat at home using in denial until my mother called on October 30, 2019. She was yelling and telling me to stay away from her because she just got her bank statement from my dad's trust fund. She asked why I stole that much money, and then she asked if I was doing drugs. Something was different this time, and I cried out, "Yes, mom, I'm on drugs and it's bad. Real bad. And I need help." Into detox I went. It was a state-funded detox, so I was scared out of my wits.

After 2 days of being on Suboxone, I laughed. I could not believe that I had laughed and meant it. I felt it. I was living again. I began feeling all sorts of feelings. I felt like I was myself again. I didn't have any cravings. Every day, for the past 15 years, all I thought about was getting money for drugs, doing drugs, counting drugs, and ordering more drugs. It was like I wasn't a slave anymore. I was free. I could think clearly, and I noticed that I didn't have pain from my Crohn's Disease. My depression wasn't present.

I've been on this amazing medication, Suboxone, since October 2019. I attend NA meetings, and I have a sponsor. I like the support of other addicts. It makes me feel normal. Well, I feel like a normal recovering addict. My life is 100% better because I'm living it. I'm learning how to live again without drugs.

- Dawn D Providence, RI

What Does it Mean to be in Recovery?

In this book, we use the term "recovery," but what does it really mean. One way to describe it is to compare it with someone who has cancer. The recovery process is a lot like being "in remission."

What being in recovery from addiction means is that you are no longer suffering from the drug addiction, but you're aren't quite out of the woods. Unlike other types of diseases, there is no drug that can promise to heal you from addiction. There's no cure; just treatment.

Being in recovery means you are actively taking part in programs to help you overcome the chemical, psychological, social, and environmental aspects of addiction. Like overcoming any other form of disease, you are actively fighting the challenges of addiction each and every day. It takes focus and determination.

Take it One Day at a Time

Taking on addiction is a battle. Most battles aren't won in a day, week, or even a month. Don't let this intimidate you. All you have to do is take it one day at a time and remember that each day brings with it the opportunity to win another battle. You will be faced with temptations. You will have days where you'll think, "This completely sucks. Why don't I just start using again?" By winning the daily battle, you can focus on winning the week, the month, the year, and ultimately, **your life**.

What is it Like Being in Recovery?

When you are early in recovery, taking it one day at a time might be too overwhelming. You might have to take it an hour, a minute, or even seconds at a time. Recovery is a process, and you have to experience it deeply to appreciate its meaning.

When you are in recovery, you:

- Feel a kinship to those who are also in recovery

- Make decisions based on how it could impact your recovery

- Adjust friendships and relationships based on how they could affect recovery

- Never let down your guard

There is no part of your life that recovery will not touch. Your recovery is a daily reminder to appreciate what you have. You may find that sharing time with others in recovery and talking to them about their experiences can soothe you and ignite empathy that you can also give to yourself. It's important to treat yourself kindly and generously while you are in recovery, for as long as it may serve you and your process.

Relapse During Recovery

One important thing to know about the recovery process of addiction is that you will need to make changes to your lifestyle. Recovery simply isn't about removing substances from your life; it also means making changes in your life that initially led to substance abuse and dependence. And this can be quite difficult, which is why relapsing is a common step in the recovery process.

Relapsing

What Happens if You Fail?

The success rate of Medication-Assisted Therapies is in the 50-75% range. This means that there is no guarantee that you will succeed the first time around. The important thing is to not give up.

If you stumble, we're not going to kick you out of the program. As counselors, we recognize that the chemicals in your brain are fighting against you. It's a tough battle.

Let's say you go six months without using and you slip up. Your next goal should be to see if you can go seven months next time. To equate it to football, it's like moving up to the goal post each time until you finally reach that goal.

Recovery Connection's Philosophy

At Recovery Connection, we understand that the path to recovery is hardly ever a straight line. There are hurdles, twists, and turns. That is just a realistic perspective. You will have temptations. There are days where you will need to use all your strength and resources to not go the easy way and begin using drugs again.

It is absolutely a learning curve. As counselors, we learn from every patient we meet because everyone's path is different and comes with its own set of unique challenges. We want you to overcome the temptation to hide things from us. If you slip and use again, we are not going to yell at you. What we will do is ask you what you learned from the experience, and we will let you know we're happy you returned to us. Let us figure out a way to better you so you are less likely to slip up in the future. Let's use what happened and build from it, from the perspective of a counselor and as a patient.

We understand. It's part of our innate being to want what we shouldn't have. The goal of Medication-Assisted Therapy is to eventually make your days **not** using better than any of the days when you were using. Now, if you come in for opiate addiction treatment and then you start showing up with a new drug in your system each week, that is something we will need to address. We will need to figure out why you are using other substances. And that's the importance of continuing to come in for counseling so we can find that out.

We want to know why you are putting yourself in those types of situations. As counselors, we will want to reach into our toolkit and look at our resources to see if maybe a higher level of care would be appropriate for you. That's the importance of continuing counseling. It's not that you make a mistake but that you gain something from the mistake. Turn a negative moment into a positive one and see how you can move forward.

Shift Your Environment

During recovery, you might want to consider changing your environment, even if that simply means moving apartments. You might also want to block and/or delete your dealer contacts. That will help separate yourself from those influences. If you know other people that are doing those drugs, it is always a good idea to try to separate yourself from those kinds of people.

One thing we've discovered in our years as former users and now as counselors and doctors is that users devote so much of their day to searching for, acquiring, and using drugs. This means that once we put them on buprenorphine, they all of a sudden have a lot more time and money on their hands. The key is to use that time and money wisely.

Cycle of Recovery

What happens to most individuals in treatment is that they will cycle. What this means is that they will begin using, hit a wall, seek treatment, (mistakenly) believe they have their life sorted out, start using again, and the process repeats ad nauseum. You might start the process of getting treatment for a few weeks before you begin to say,

"This sucks. I'm going to start using again. It's just simpler. I don't want to deal with this. I'm not ready to change my life." So, you'll go back to using. Later, you'll most likely say, "This sucks. How do I turn my life around?" The second time around you might make a more concerted effort to get help. And this time, you will likely stick with it for a bit longer. You might even stay with treatment for six months or even a year.

It's important to stick with treatments. Because when you get off the routine of going into treatment on a continuous basis, it almost feels like starting over. Of the thousands of patients we've treated over the years at Recovery Connection, only a handful were instances where they were able to run through the program without falling off momentarily. What we mean by straight through is that they were addicted to heroin, Oxycodone, Percocet, or some other opiate and they were able to go through treatment and have stayed clean after the fact.

The Reality of Recovery and Relapse

Recovery is a battle, a saga, a marathon — whatever phrase that describes a long, arduous journey. That is what you can expect while undergoing buprenorphine therapy. Drug addiction doesn't care about your age, gender, or background. It is an equal opportunity destroyer. Pick any treatment center in the world and you may find yourself sitting across from a homeless person, lawyer, doctor, high school student, or a CEO.

Likewise, everyone at these clinics receives the same treatment. As we mentioned earlier, those with drug addiction have a 60% comorbidity for mental illness, which means that most patients have underlying issues that should be treated in order to break the cycle of substance abuse.

At Recovery Connection, we work to find underlying issues that could cause someone to relapse into substance abuse. Some of the most common causes are mental illness, grief (loss of a loved one), PTSD, or it may even be an environmental issue with home life or work.

Researchers found the greatest risk factors for women who relapsed were withdrawal symptoms, depression and post-traumatic stress disorder. For men, the most significant risk factors included multiple substance use disorders and a history of conduct disorder, a behavioral disorder in which the basic rights of others or rules are violated. Younger age was identified as a major risk factor for both men and women relapsing as well.

"These results suggest that women would particularly benefit from treatments that aggressively address withdrawal symptoms with appropriate medications and cognitive-behavioral approaches," said lead author **Jordan Davis**, an assistant professor at the USC Suzanne Dworak-Peck School of Social Work and Associate Director of the **USC Center for Artificial Intelligence in Society**.

He further commented on the best approaches for men by stating, "In contrast, men would likely benefit most from cognitive-behavioral and mutual-help interventions that directly target substance use behaviors and support the development of pro-social behaviors."

Future relapse prevention treatment research should explore ways to mitigate these specific and different vulnerabilities for men and women. In addition, Davis believes machine learning approaches should be more widely integrated into addiction research to better understand the complexities of how demographic, psychological and behavioral variables may increase the odds of relapse.

"Our approach allowed us to look at different trajectories of relapse. We're able to show, for example, if you're an adolescent female who has high criminal justice involvement, this is your risk of relapse," said another study author **John Prindle**, Research Assistant Professor at the USC Suzanne Dworak-Peck School of Social Work. "Ultimately, machine learning is the future of modeling and understanding data in addiction science," emphasized Prindle.[15]

Counseling During Recovery

As you go through the process of recovery, something strange will likely happen to you. You will begin to feel like your normal self — the self before you started using opiates. You will discover the joy of feeling like you are in the present moment. You will also experience what it is like to not have to constantly worry about where your next fix will come from (or being arrested). Another thing that will happen is that all of those thoughts, feelings, and emotions you've locked away will begin to emerge. This is the moment that you will soon understand the value of counseling in Medication-Assisted Treatment.

When you are able to incorporate counseling into your recovery process, you can start to look at the deeper issues that led you to drugs in the first place. This is invaluable because dealing with the root of the addiction allows the combination of MAT and the emotional treatment to encourage full recovery. The reason is, when you no longer need a substance to address issues in your life, the desire for them may decrease.

In the next chapter, we will get more specific with the research behind the value of counseling as well as the positive results experienced by patients using the Recovery Connection treatment method.

Chapter 10
Recovery Connection is About Connecting

John's* Story

My addiction was to hydrocodone, oxycodone and OxyContin exclusively because that was readily available to me, and I liked how they made me feel at first. I was more productive, cheerful and generally a better person – or so I thought. After a few years, it was becoming painfully clear that I was no longer getting any psychological benefit from my drug use. I was simply managing my withdrawals from pill to pill. My life consisted of waking up, seeking drugs until I found them and then starting all over the next day. When I couldn't find my drugs or ran short of cash, the world would quickly start crashing down around me.

I am by no means a material person, but everyone has something in this world that is precious to them. All I had left of my grandfather was a gold watch he had given me before he died. No matter how bad off I had gotten over the years, I held onto that watch, as it always gave me great comfort. I had it in my pocket the day I got married; the day I was in a mine cave-in and thought my life was over; and every other important junction of my life.

About one year ago, I found myself low on cash while waiting for my tax refund. I had a chance to score a large number of pills and save some cash in the long run. I pawned the watch for the pills with every intention of getting it back with my refund. Like a true junkie, I never got the watch out of hock. I spent the refund on more pills. I lost more than a watch that day, I lost my self-respect, and

---

* Name changed to protect privacy

I knew for sure that my self-control was all but gone as well. Addiction makes all of us do things we would never have dreamed of.

Even though it took another year of addiction before I had the resolve to do something, the fact that I had traded the most valuable thing to me on Earth for a handful of pills still haunts me to this day. I would give anything to have it back, but I know that it will never be. I became so sick of my life that I cut ties with my dealers in a manner that would never allow me to return. I was determined to put a stop to this or die trying.

Three days into withdrawals, I was so lost and depressed. I started searching the internet for anything that could help me. I had used a lot of methadone off the street, but I knew that was not a direction that I wanted. In-patient rehab was an absolute last resort that would have destroyed my job and hurt those around me. I was going to beat this thing or take my own life if I couldn't. I then came across Recovery Connection. People there gave me direction. I found an excellent doctor with a real understanding of addiction and Suboxone therapy. No games, no lies and no blind enthusiasm. He clearly explained what Sub does, and told me, in no uncertain terms, that the success or failure of this treatment was up to me. Suboxone could only help me cure my addiction in the long run if I was determined to do so.

In terms of trading one addiction for another, my doctor explained it like this: "You are trading addictive behavior for medical behavior, and this therapy will give you the chance to address the true causes of your addiction." He was correct about the behavior; if the drugs didn't kill me, then the people and places I had frequented eventually would have.

I've realized that even though Suboxone has given me a new chance and I'm on the right path for recovery, there are some things my addiction has changed forever. I've been in jail and lost valued relationships over drugs but selling that damn watch will be with me until the day I die.

- John J Seekonk, MA

Breaking Down the Walls and Rediscovering the Real You

Most of us are not open about our addiction. It's not an aspect of life we willingly share with others (that is, unless we are around other people who have substance use disorder as well). During the course of your addiction, you've learned to build up a façade to protect yourself from judgement and scrutiny.

In all likelihood, by the time you enter into a drug treatment program, that phony image you've created for yourself is already starting to show signs of cracking. Despite the walls you've put up, your counselor is your confidante and your partner. They will help you to transition into a new reality and help you build a foundation for a better you.

Open the Flood Gates

What this also means is that all those emotions you've bottled up over the years will begin to pour out. Don't be surprised if the flood gates open and you find yourself overwhelmed with a bevy of emotions — all of that has been bottled up under pressure for a long time. Your counselor will help you to sort through your emotions and put things into perspective.

There will be aspects of yourself that will be difficult to confront. Don't worry. Your counselor isn't naive; they know that addiction can make people do things they later regret. Your counselor will be there to help you organize your thoughts, ask questions, answer questions, and help you to build positive coping mechanisms when you are confronted with urges/cravings in the future.

Counseling is About Community

One of the reasons those with addiction are closest to others with addictions is because it serves as sort of a community through shared experiences. The same is true for those going through the recovery process. You should feel like you are part of a community, working together to achieve a common goal.

Like many other types of MAT facilities, Recovery Connection provides a variety of services that help people reconnect with themselves and others and find their place in the community. There are plenty of outreach programs operated by those who are also in recovery. These community services are aimed at helping people find jobs and other resources that bring much-needed stability.

Building a Recovery Plan

One of the beneficial aspects of counseling is that, together with your counselor, you will develop short- and long-term treatment plans. These are specifically tailored for you, so if you feel uncomfortable with any aspect of the plan, be sure to inform your counselor.

To help create your treatment plan, the counselor will want to know your backstory and how you became addicted to your drug of choice. The counselor may ask you questions such as:

- Did you become dependent on opioids due to a doctor's prescriptions following an injury?

- Did you climb the ladder of other recreational drugs until you discovered opioids?

- Do you have friends and family that currently use opioids or other recreational drugs?

- Do you have friends or family that can positively influence your recovery?

Your counselor will also want to know about your social environment. They will likely ask you about where you live, whether you have stable housing, and if you have support from family and friends. Where do you usually get your drugs? Will you be able to stay away from your dealer? (Many times, your dealer is a friend or family member).

Comorbidities

As we discussed earlier in the book, there are a whole host of psychological disorders that make drugs such as opioids appealing. Opiates temporarily elevate dopamine, which relieves depression. Drugs like heroin, Percocet, and other opioids can create a temporary illusion of stability in those suffering from psychological disorders. The National Institute on Drug Abuse lists several psychological disorders that tend to cause people to seek drugs for relief. These include:

- Depression

- Bipolar disorder

- Attention-Deficit Hyperactivity Disorder (ADHD)

- Psychotic illness

- Post-Traumatic Stress Disorder (PTSD)

- Borderline Personality Disorder (BPD)

- Antisocial Personality Disorder

If you believe that you may be suffering from one of these illnesses, then you should know that going through a drug treatment program will help you with addiction, but the compounding factor that led you to addiction will still be there on the other side. Therefore, it's important that you receive counseling and treatment for any psychological disorder you may be experiencing. You might also want to look into dual diagnosis treatments, which tackle psychological and addiction disorders simultaneously.

It is estimated that upwards of 60% of individuals who use illicit substances also have mental illness as a comorbidity. This means that 60% of patients with opiate issues also have an underlying mental health issue.

Most patients don't use drugs because their lives are perfect. At many treatment facilities, including Recovery Connection, we will look at whether there are underlying factors (such as PTSD or depression), which should also be evaluated so we can include that in the treatment plan.

You Lead the Treatment

At centers such as Recovery Connection, the patient is in the driver's seat. When you come to us for treatment, we are not going to dictate every aspect of your treatment. We want patients to participate as much as possible and to be honest with the counselors.

We want to inspire you, motivate you, and keep you involved in the treatment process as much as possible. So long as you continue to show up wanting and trying to fight for your own recovery, we will be there right alongside you. We will continue to help you find a treatment path that works best for you.

Counselors and doctors want patients to be open and honest. Likewise, the counselors and doctors will be transparent about the treatment process. We also want you to participate. By being active in the program, we can better assess and respond to your needs, improving your chances of success.

The Importance of Counseling

Many counselors and those who have gone through the Medication-Assisted Therapy process will tell you that while the medication is important in achieving stability, it is really the counseling that helps patients maintain a life free of illicit substances. Even as you are chemically stabilized by the buprenorphine, you will still be challenged by your environment and your own actions since opiate dependency is a recurring disease.

The counseling portion of treatment will likely far outlast the medication part of treatment. Counseling is here to make sure that when you do hit those bumps in the road, the resources and support that come about through counseling will be there for you. When you do seek out a Medication-Assisted Treatment facility, one of the questions you could ask them is, "How long does counseling last?" The correct answer should be, "As long as necessary."

At Recovery Connection, counseling is included whenever a patient checks in for their regular Suboxone prescription. Making that connection with a counselor helps patients stay on track with their treatment plans.

The Counselor

During your initial visit, you will also speak with a counselor. The counselor will look over your paperwork as well as the treatment plan set by the doctor. The role of the counselor is to essentially guide your path and ensure you are taking your prescribed medications correctly (whether that's Suboxone or some other type of therapy).

When it comes to counseling, it doesn't matter if you have an appointment. Someone should be there for you to discuss whatever issues you may be going through. The doctor and counselor both want you to succeed, and that means getting off to a good start.

There's Always an Open Door

Most treatment facilities have an open-door policy. If there's something urgent that you feel you need to discuss, the facility should be able to arrange counseling or consultations with the doctor in a timely manner. This is true for Recovery Connection Centers of America.

The Mental Battle

Medication-Assisted Therapies can take you halfway to where you want to be — a life free of addiction and free from the urge to use illicit substances. Medication makes it easier, but you will likely have a mental battle ahead of you. Speaking openly, freely, and often with your counselor can help you to get the upper hand in the fight. During the treatment process, you should have at least one person (even if it's just the counselor) that will be there to listen.

What is My Future?

There is no set timeline of how long you should be on buprenorphine or go through counseling. All treatment plans are personalized to meet the person's unique needs. Even after the medication part of therapy is over, you will likely still have the same issues that led you to becoming dependent on substances. Even if you feel good in your situation currently and your relationships are going well, a few months from now you could lose your job or be faced with some other obstacle that might tempt you back to using. The point is, no matter how good you feel right now, you will be faced with obstacles that will test you. Counseling serves as a safety net or support during those times when things aren't going ideal.

Once you complete the buprenorphine stage of therapy, you should continue the counseling portion. Even though you'll no longer be using, you might experience some bumps in the road or find it difficult to handle the cravings. Maintaining that contact with a counselor can be very helpful in working through those cravings.

Starting to Feel Normal

Many patients that begin treatment do so because they are afraid of entering into withdrawals. When they start buprenorphine, they discover that not only are they not going through withdrawals, but they catch a glimpse of what "normal" feels like again. They feel comfortable and clear-headed. They catch sight of what their future can be: free of illicit substances. This is part of the problem.

Remember this: If you ever go to an AA meeting, you will likely hear someone introduce themselves by saying, "Hello, I'm XXXX. I've been an alcoholic for 30 years, but I stopped drinking 25 years ago." The reason for this is that we all must recognize the potential to relapse. We are all fighting something that doesn't disappear with time. It gets better each year, but it doesn't disappear completely. The treatments and counseling you receive while going through the process will help cure the symptoms, but the potential to use again will always be there.

The good news is that you can stay on buprenorphine for as long as you'd like. If you'd like to indefinitely have your opioid receptors plugged up with a very minor dose of buprenorphine, as counselors, we will endorse that if that's what you need to do to stay clean — even if it just means taking a .5 milligram dose. We've had people say, "I want to stay at this level because my life has improved so much from where I was at."

If you've been using heroin for two or three years, you shouldn't expect to come off Suboxone within a matter of months. This would simply not be a good outcome since you are not chemically and psychological ready for that kind of transition. It doesn't even have to be heroin; you may have been involved in some type of injury and you became addicted to doctor-prescribed medications, which led you to take more than prescribed, and suddenly you're searching for more opiates. Either way, giving yourself time for treatment even if you start feeling normal is essential to long-term recovery.

What Now?

While this book has not been an exhaustive compilation of all the information concerning opioid addiction and treatment options, the goal was to give you enough accurate information so you can make a decision that is sound and well-informed. All of the staff here at Recovery Connection have had some sort of experience with addiction, whether that be personally or secondary. Either way, these experiences give us a level of passion and knowledge that allow us to treat the entire patient. We aren't just looking to get people on medication and send them on their way. We want people to be fully treated – physically, mentally, emotionally, and spiritually.

As you've seen from the testimonials that were throughout this book, we have seen both sides of addiction. We've seen our patients come in with severe issues that made them feel like their life was out of control. But, at the same time, we've seen these same people take their lives back and start living again.

This doesn't have to be a mere fantasy or wish. It can be a place to start. And really, as we discussed in the stages of change, you will overcome the hardest part by simply admitting that you need help and then asking for it. Whether you are local to one of our offices in the New England area or not, we welcome you to reach out to receive information, support and hope.

Contact us at:
www.drughelp.com
(877) 557-3155

Helpful Resources

Substance Abuse and Mental Health Services Administration (U.S. Department of Health & Human Services)

https://www.samhsa.gov/find-help/national-helpline

1-800-662-4357 (1-800-662-HELP)

Endnotes

[1] Joyce Frieden, Washington Editor, MedPage Today June 1, 2021

[2] https://www.kipu.health/emr-blog/treatment-trends-for-2021-and-beyond/

[3] https://www.kipu.health/emr-blog/millennium-health-an-inside-look-at-drug-testing

[4] https://jamanetwork.com/journals/jamanetworkopen/fullarticle/2776442

[5] Copeland, W. E., Keeler, G., Angold, A., & Costello, E. J. (2007). Traumatic events and posttraumatic stress in childhood. *Archives of General Psychiatry, 64*, 577-584. https://doi.org/10.1001/archpsyc.64.5.577

[6] https://www.samhsa.gov/sites/default/files/aatod_2018_final.pdf

[7] https://www.ncbi.nlm.nih.gov/pmc/articles/PMC3681508/

[8] Nahin RL. Estimates of pain prevalence and severity in adults: United States, 2012. J Pain. 2015;16:769–780

[9] (Vowles KE, McEntee ML, Julnes PS, Frohe T, Ney JP, van der Goes DN. Rates of opioid misuse, abuse, and addiction in chronic pain: a systematic review and data synthesis. Pain. 2015;156:569–576)

[10] https://www.mayoclinic.org/diseases-conditions/prescription-drug-abuse/in-depth/how-opioid-addiction-occurs/art-20360372

[11] https://www.drugabuse.gov/drug-topics/health-consequences-drug-misuse/mental-health-effects

[12] https://s3.amazonaws.com/academia.edu.documents/46826667/Opioid_Addiction_Changes_Cerebral_Blood

[13] https://baartprograms.com/5-ways-opioids-impact-relationships-with-loved-ones/

[14] DiClemente, C.C. Motivational interviewing and the stages of change. In: Miller, W.R., and Rollnick, S., eds. Motivational Interviewing: Preparing People To Change Addictive Behavior. New York: Guilford Press, 1991. Pp. 191-202

[15] https://news.usc.edu/182665/risk-factors-opioid-relapse-men-women-usc-research/